THE POWER OF POSITIVE STRETCHING

by Evelyn Loewendahl

Ward Ritchie Press
Pasadena, California

Acknowledgments

Sincere thanks to my many patients over the years, who taught me the preciousness of good health; to my students—young, eager, and unknowledge-able—who showed the delightful quality of excite-ment in new learning; to my professional colleagues and fellow clinicians, who demonstrated the un-relenting hope even in the dimmest hours; to my many friends for their patience and comments in reading the manuscript; to my devoted typist Evelyn Shepard; to all of you, my deep appreciation for help and encouragement.

Contents

Introduction

Intro

The story of man's ability to move is the story of increasingly complex physical development. Eons ago, the salamander slithered along, propelling its body forward with a swish of its powerful tail. This type of locomotion required the expansion and contraction of the belly tissues and, although primitive, was efficient for the salamander's survival.

After millions of years, four-legged animals evolved, and with them a more advanced type of locomotion developed. Because these animals were more complex, they moved more efficiently and were able to perform a greater variety of movements. Running, leaping, climbing, and trotting—all of which took muscle strength and endurance—developed. In the case of animals like the greyhound and cheetah, the structure evolved to where the animals were able to attain tremendous speed.

When two-legged animals came into existence—for birds this was about 135 million years later—the actual efficiency of movement dropped. The forelegs evolved into wings, which enabled the animal to fly, but on the ground the bird's movement was so slow that some species were endangered to the point of extinction.

In man the forelegs, or arms, became even less efficient than the wings of the bird. They aided balance in walking, but their absence did not alter the gait significantly. The legs alone carried the burden for walking, standing, and moving.

Why man ever stood up remains a mystery. Four-legged creatures move more efficiently. They can maintain their balance as they run, leap, or jump, and they can climb easily, freely, and efficiently, all without using any pills, ointments, or heating pads later to soothe sore bodies. The erect torso of man has exacted its price, and up to now modern living has not helped to improve the efficiency and comfort of man's structure in motion.

In terms of human history, we discovered only yesterday that our mobility could be maintained with a unique do-it-yourself program. But in terms of today's knowledge, the news media will tell us more about getting to the moon or even Mars than they will about a simple program to take care of our bodies, to prevent and undo the premature breakdown of body parts.

And that is the reason for this book. Although medical science made the discoveries, no one took the trouble to get the word to you, who can best use this knowledge to keep your body youthful, mobile, and free.

There are many books available that deal with exercise programs designed primarily to improve man's structure and function. These deal with muscle strengthening, such as the Canadian fitness manual; isotonic programs; and cardiac fitness, such as aerobics in jogging. There are also many books on yoga, which is a stretch program, but one that is highly complicated and in need of intensive modification for general use. *The Power of Positive Stretching,* however, is a fresh and unique body-conditioning book, one that departs sharply from traditional concepts of an exercise program. It does not deal with muscles but concentrates instead on connective tissue and its influence on our ability to move freely.

Connective tissue is the most widespread material in our physical structure; it fills all spaces, corners, and crevices. But more important, it is the substance that wraps each individual muscle fiber and encases the whole muscle bundle. It further extends to form a tough, elastic attachment to a bone, called a tendon. Other connective structures, including the very tough bands at the base of the skull and the base of the spinal column, are known as ligaments.

Whether a layer covering some organ or an attachment to a bony protuberance, connective tissue is the substance that determines our range of motion —our ability to move freely, to bend, twist, and turn easily. How far can you fling your arm? Your leg? How far can you bend forward? Can you turn your head all the way to the side or only part of the way? These are all ranges of motion associated with our ability to move, and they are determined by the factor of stretchability.

Through aging and inactivity, connective tissue will shorten and lose its elasticity, leaving you vulnerable to potential physical disability. Through a series of stretches, however, elasticity can be restored and maintained, freeing you from stiffness and pain and improving your mental and physical health.

In this book you will learn about connective tissue and how to keep it supple. You will learn about the nature of the body structure and why you can improve body function through stretching. This knowledge not only will enhance your understanding of the human form, but will give you the simple tools for correcting and improving the condition of your body.

Judging from the billions of dollars spent on pills, medications, and devices that promote relief, millions of Americans suffer from body aches and stiffness, and a body program like this that provides relatively fast relief has something valuable to offer many people. Practically everyone in modern society could benefit, since our lifestyle forces cramped living on us, whether we spend our time commuting to work or relaxing in front of the television. To stretch out the body, to counteract the debilitating shortening of the body bindings, is the main goal of this book.

The stretch routines detailed here not only are simple but are directed to specific body parts. For example, if tension, tightness, and stiffness are located in the neck region, a stretch is provided for that part of the body. If stiffness is located in the upper spine, that area and that area only is relaxed through thoracic elongation. It is entirely possible for one part of the body to be completely flexible while another part is stiff. Each side of the body can be tested, and stiffness can be further pinpointed at the precise segment of the physical structure that needs attention.

It is important to conserve energy not only in the environment but in ourselves and, happily, the stretches don't call for extreme exertion. They can be done in a reclining position, and this relaxed pose (see Figure A) has great appeal for older people, those who must restrict their activity, and those who dislike sweat-and-toil exercises.

Other stretches, however, call for more vigorous action, and these have great appeal for dancers, athletes, young persons, and those individuals who enjoy being very active and feeling alive.

For the depressed or tired individual, lack of energy for getting started can actually be alleviated by the simplest stretch, which triggers deeper breathing. The increased oxygen intake breaks the cycle of fatigue and lack of energy, and the freer the joint, the greater the stimulus for oxygen intake.

It is well known that feelings of freedom, well-being, relief, and relaxation transmit themselves to the physical realm, and consequently, professionals are learning that lack of body tension is directly concomitant to good mental as well as physical health. We are all aware of the need to move in order to let off steam. Built-up tensions must be released, or severe damage to the psyche results. The pot smasher and the dish thrower are all expressing the need to release emotional tension.

Exercise, however, is a much more harmless way. Grab a racket, run a mile, or stretch your way to emotional calm. When Dwight D. Eisenhower was supreme commander of the armed forces in Europe, he too was under unbearable emotional tension before the invasion of Normandy. But he walked daily, played golf, and rode horseback, and whenever his staff showed signs of stress, he prescribed physical activity. He did not send them to the staff psychiatrist because the physical route relieved their tensions more quickly. Primitive societies also recognize the need for physical outlets to promote emotional health and consequently incorporate yelling, violent dancing, drum pounding, etc. into their rituals.

A few things should be pointed out about the effectiveness of this new preventive modality—the stretch. How to motivate you is the biggest challenge of all. I know that I will win you over if you are

FIGURE A.
The relaxed position, with
the knees up and the feet
flat on the floor, creates
good alignment of the
spinal column. With the
body at ease and the hips
flat, stretch both arms back
flat on the floor. Your arms,
shoulders, ribs, and waist
will receive a gentle stretch
in this relaxed position.

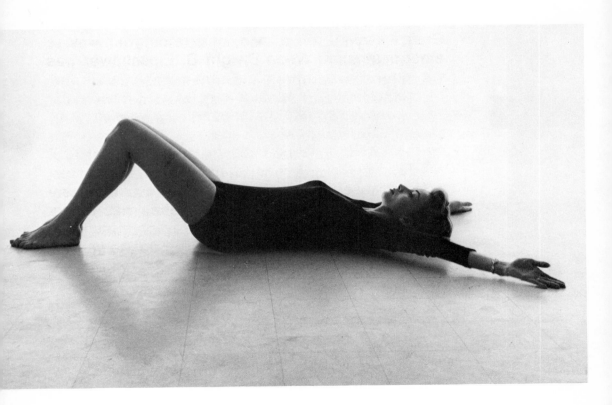

aware, alert, and intelligent enough to realize that you are given only one body and that taking good care of it makes it last.

Sudden fears or recently acquired knowledge wear off quickly, but once you begin to feel great —to feel alive—to feel younger than you have in years—your joy will not disappear. You will realize that it just feels too good to quit. Eventually you will even reach the point where you miss the stretching if you don't do it.

I can lose your interest, however, because:

- The record shows that all health spas lose their initial enthusiasts within the first six months; there is an 80 percent drop-out rate.
- Once you achieve complete range of motion, especially if you do it rather quickly, you may forget to stretch and rationalize away your body's deterioration. It may take a severe stress warning to remind you of the value of continuing your stretches.
- The American people in general have a reputation for being poorly disciplined. Even one stretch a day has to be put into a routine that is repeated over and over again to make it a habit. Whether you are in a space capsule or a high-rise apartment complex, the problem of daily stretching is the same.

Perhaps the most important thing to recognize is that stretching is a scientific tool. It is a cheap one, readily available to everyone as a health measure if we take the time to learn a few simple rules, techniques, and applications.

So I ask you to join a goal-oriented program that promises far more dividends than any other investment you can make. The modern trend is to anticipate health disasters rather than wait for deterioration and, fortunately, many people today are taking preventive measures. Call it holistic medicine, aging with a future, getting healthier as you grow older, or whatever. The cost is a little effort, a little learning, and modest performance.

1 Body ABCs

Body
ABCs

In their space capsules, our pioneering U.S. astronauts were stuffed into an area no bigger than the front seat of a sports car. These space pioneers and all subsequent astronauts were in top physical form before launching and, aware of their need to maintain good body function, ground specialists prepared a set of rubberized cords that the astronauts could use for exercising in space. But the factor of confinement was not considered in these initial explorations, and in less than one week, the astronauts were plagued with a stiffness that the strongest muscles and most powerful endurance factors on earth and in space could not alleviate. No wonder they complained in one of their conversations with ground control:

Astronaut: We're beginning to feel the effects of being confined—we're getting stiff.

Ground Control: Maybe you ought to open the door and stretch a little.

Astronaut: I'd sure like to.

The confinement in the initial flights was so debilitating that preparations for the moon trips included experiments with freer garments in place of the heavy space suits so that the body would be free to move and stretch. In the trips to the moon, man ultimately traveled in his underwear and wore the confining space suit only when he left the capsule and walked in space.

Believe it or not, the stresses and strains suffered by your body under day-in and day-out, year-in and year-out use can result in the same stiffness that the astronauts experienced. Sitting in front of television for days without getting out, or lying in bed for a prolonged period has the same effect. Whether we are talking about man on earth or man in space, the body needs to be mobile. This is simply part of our physical inheritance and is based on a long history of physical structure that needs to function in motion.

The bindings of the body in anatomical terms are known as connective tissue. This is living fiber that binds our muscles, organs, and joints together. It can be elongated and also shortened, and it is these basic qualities that make its proper functioning crucial.

The effect of body bindings on our general health has been so recently revealed that we are just beginning to appreciate the importance of their capacity to *yield.* Most of the minor ailments and body stress suffered today are caused by body bindings that cannot yield easily, readily, fully, and comfortably. The flexibility of the points where each binding is attached will indicate whether the tissue is yielding, or tight and unyielding.

A hundred years ago in a society requiring more physical labor and less sitting in confined quarters, there was no need to focus on the importance of body bindings and the role they play in health. Daily chores stretched them enough to keep the body flexible and free.

Ever since Greece staged the first Olympic games, athletes have known the value of flexibility. The Greek civilization stressed physical perfection in harmony with spiritual development, and the importance of concentrating on keeping the body moving freely became clear when civilization began fencing us in.

For centuries poor posture was regarded merely as part of a slovenly appearance and the cause of a few minor mechanical failures; most popular books stressed exercise to keep muscles well-formed and strong.

But lesser-known but more expert pioneers in the field of body mechanics, such as Dr. R. F. Ober of Harvard, a real early pioneer; Dr. Harvey Billig of Stanford; and Dr. Charles Leroy Lowman, founder of the Los Angeles Orthopedic Hospital, now have attracted our attention. Scholarly body professionals have learned the value of the explorations of these early medical specialists. They and other top authorities explored the relationship between the excessive contraction (overshortening) of connective tissue bindings and common body-disabling conditions. They discovered that if the overshortening continued, one could develop many physical problems.

In London at St. Thomas' Hospital, Dr. James B. Mennell developed mechanical stretching techniques to relieve the stiffness from which many patients were suffering.

Dr. George Hassard, specialist in physical medicine and rehabilitation at the University of Oklahoma, writes in his book *Elongation Treatment of Low Back Pain,* "It is now established that body bindings have the quality of contractility and elasticity that other body tissues have." And, according to *Postural Fitness,* a book by Drs. Lowman and Carl Haven Young, "It is obvious that it is necessary to stretch before improved body alignment can be obtained. Limbering-up exercises improve all metabolic processes."

Increasingly, medical doctors are agreeing that some type of scientific stretching will minimize the stiffness associated with normal aging. At the same time, it will keep a person relaxed, in good condition, and free from minor body irritations. These procedures have been successful in relieving headaches, backaches, and foot pains, and now you can loosen your own body bindings by simple stretches. Perhaps most important, you can prevent premature overstiffness and avoid the aged look of tight, bent-over bodies.

This material took shape out of personal experience with patients in a research and treatment program. First, there were the haunting groans and tears of patients often doubled over with pain. Then, after stretch treatments, their sighs of relief. Next came the evidence of the role that taut tissue plays in creating stiffness and pain, documented in the study of thousands of post-polio patients at the California Institute of Technology in Pasadena, where I participated in neuromuscular research in a treatment and testing program for post-poliomyelitis cases.

Muscle imbalance, the result of nerve damage, leaves many persons with stiffness and immobile joints. The problem—to free the joints in order to restore mobility—must be alleviated before any muscle strengthening can take place. Frequent observation of the need to restore joint flexibility has proven the primary importance of relieving tissue tightness. In many instances, the mere relief of joint stiffness gives muscles a far better opportunity to function.

Inelastic bindings are as great a hazard to restoration of limb function as weakened muscles are and are equally, sometimes more, hazardous for normal muscles not damaged by any injury or disease because there is no question that restricted body bindings deplete the power of muscles. I have examined countless young people in a posture fitness program who could not easily raise their legs off the floor while face down on all fours (see Figure 1). When the bindings in the fore part of their hips were loosened through stretches, however, the back hip muscles could contract further, and this enabled the patients to raise their legs higher. A much more normal functional ability was thus restored.

Years of inactivity, which produce tight body bindings, will cause any muscles to deteriorate, and this might lead to the false conclusion that the muscles themselves are weak. By releasing the bindings, you will restore the ability of the muscle to contract to its fullest potential and, consequently, when the muscle is free and unbound, it automatically restores its function—namely contracting and releasing—and it will no longer be held within a restricted range of motion.

In college therapy courses I have demonstrated the role that stiffness plays in muscle loss by tying a student's forearm in a wooden splint for three days, then measuring the circumference just below the elbow. It usually measures one-quarter inch less than it did before splinting, when it had been free and unbound. Without injury or disease, then, merely from lack of use and immobility, the muscles of

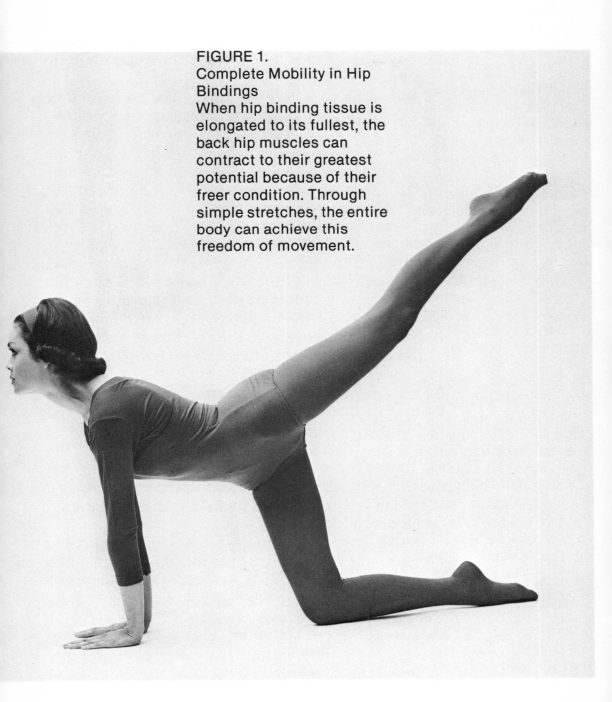

FIGURE 1.
Complete Mobility in Hip
Bindings
When hip binding tissue is
elongated to its fullest, the
back hip muscles can
contract to their greatest
potential because of their
freer condition. Through
simple stretches, the entire
body can achieve this
freedom of movement.

FIGURE 2.
Test for Total Body Flexibility

Standing with your feet together, bend forward loosely, allowing your fingertips to extend as close to the floor as possible. Allow all body parts from the hips down to hang forward limply without any tension. How far are your fingertips from the floor? If you can touch the floor *with your knees straight,* your body bindings are flexible, with complete body range.

If your fingertips stop at any point between your hips and toes, however, there are tight spots in your bindings that will not let you bend forward all the way. Repeating this simple test throughout the stretch program will indicate to you how far you are progressing.

(a)

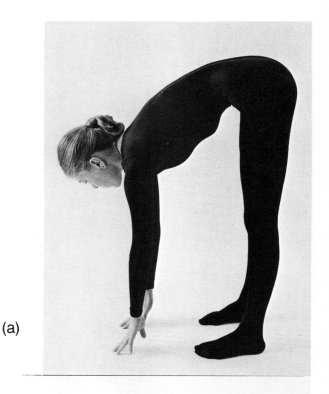

(b)

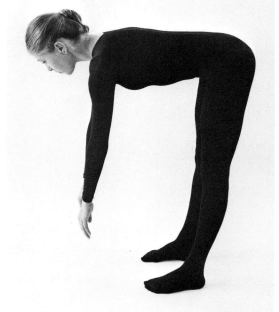

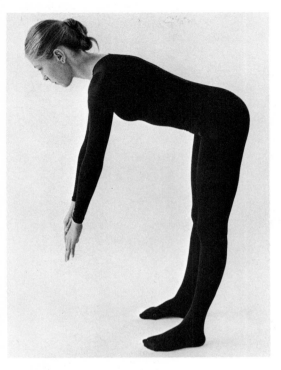

(c)

At 20 years of age, a person should be able to bend forward with his knees straight and touch the floor with his fingertips (a).

Between 30 and 40 years, it is considered normal if a person's fingertips come within three and five inches of the floor (b).

At age 50 and older, the distance between the floor and the fingertips may increase another inch and still be considered normal (c).

Some body shortening is normal with aging. The 50-year range at age 20 or 30, however, would indicate binding tightness that should be corrected.

FIGURE 3.
A Very Mild Beginning Stretch

Swing your arms high, well over your head (a). Stretch out your ribs and waistline. Surrendering your entire trunk, and your arms, neck, and shoulders, bend forward and let your arms swing through between your legs (b).

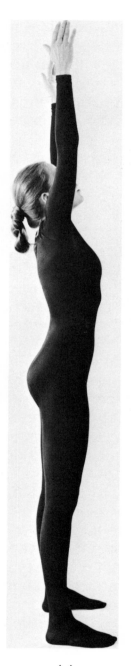

Three of these stretches morning and evening are extremely relaxing, especially when you are tired. Lying on a couch will not do nearly as much for you as these gentle body stretches.

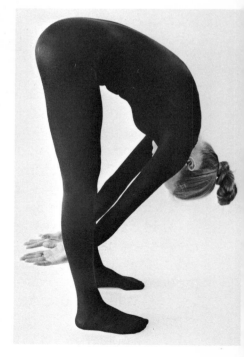

(a)   (b)

the forearm disintegrate and become stiff. In this instance arm and elbow stretches, followed by daily grips against a force every few hours, are all that is required to restore normal, satisfactory function.

Statistics show that 80 percent of those who consult a medical doctor about a "terrible pain" have common stresses and strains that will yield to self-correction. Usually all a patient needs to do is remove the restrictions that keep body bindings from yielding to free and easy motion.

Your body at 40, 50, or 60 years old is the result of how you treat it at 30 or younger. Today, medical odds favor your reaching age 65 and even beyond, but we are living longer and not liking it better, except when our bodies are comfortable—that is, unless we can move with comfort and ease and without the stress and strain that are burdensome and destroy the joy of living.

Even if you have neglected your body for 30 years, you can still improve your mobility. Living tissue is plastic and anybody's anatomy will give, no matter what his or her age. One simple stretch correctly performed every day will make a noticeable difference. And it may keep you from being a "clinic clogger"! Try the simple test for total body flexibility (see Figure 2), then try the mild beginning stretch (see Figure 3).

This simple, yet scientific primer on body stretches can make you a happier person. With self-help and brief daily application, so much can be accomplished to prevent deterioration and unwanted ills. Why not use an ounce of prevention to avoid health problems later? The goal is flexibility, and there is only one way: s–t–r–e–t–c–h.

2 The Power Within

Power
Within

June is a sewing machine operator in a garment factory. She is a steady worker with a high efficiency rating. As an employee she has one fault. Every month, for a period of three days, she is absent from work because of severe back pains during her monthly period. A posture examination shows a deeply curved-in spine.

Jack is a salesman who drives his car daily for four to five hours. His nightly shoulder pains and frequent accompanying stiff neck annoy him almost constantly.

A commuter with his arm suspended in an overhead strap is jerked to a sudden halt in a bus stop. The following day, his arm is so sore that he wonders if he broke something.

Why are Jane's monthly stress, Jack's stiff neck, and the commuter's sore arm one and the same problem? To find our answer, we must examine man's internal structure. What is man's ability to move? Does he have limits? Can anything be done to help one deal in comfort with the daily hazards of living?

These are simple questions, and we will learn the answers.

A neighbor received a large case of chinaware all the way from Hong Kong. Her eyebrows raised in pleased surprise as she lifted each unbroken piece out of the straw packing. Not one chip, crack, or break. It was almost miraculous. The delicate china had been jostled, heaved, and pounded; yet it remained whole.

Why had the dishes remained intact? The explanation to this lies in the straw packing. It *yielded.* And so it is with the bindings and "stuffings" of the human body. Your body has its own "straw" packing too, only it is known as connective tissue. This material fills all corners, crevices, and spaces inside the body, and it not only serves as a yielding inner cushion, but it covers all the organs as well. But connective tissue is more than just "packing" and covering. It also connects body structures, functioning as a rope or tie by binding muscles to bone. When it functions as such a connecting rope, it is called a ligament.

Being tied together by a ropelike substance has its advantages. Think of a juggler on the stage. He holds a small dome in his hand. On that dome he balances a small cane. On top of the small cane he places a larger cane. All the time, he shifts his feet to keep a balance. He keeps moving. On top of the second cane, the juggler places a rather large, wing-shaped bowl. Upon that he places 24 little pyramids. They sway and bend precariously, but with the quick, agile movement of his feet he keeps the objects in the air. For a grand finale, he places a solid ball on top of the 24 pyramids. The parts remain upright.

If you think of a standing person as resembling the stacked objects of the juggler, you will begin to realize the importance of balance, shifts, and mobility in the upright human body. But here the resemblance ends. Unlike the objects of the juggler, if our body parts, which are of different sizes, shapes, and weights get out of line, they do not topple to the floor. They "fall" on the body bindings. Our body bindings have such toughness and elasticity that they can take a certain amount of pressure from our body parts. They tolerate wear and tear—up to a point.

The connective "ropes" or ligaments are not fragile or easily snapped. They possess great strength and elasticity when healthy and young. They can be pounded, jostled, and assaulted, but they have their limitations. Eventually, they report their assault to the general body system. The report can vary all the way from a vague complaint of soreness to an acute attack of pain radiating from stem to stern.

Let us get back to the juggler. Notice that it was necessary to use the word *shifting* in describing the act of holding the various shapes in line. When applied to the human body, *shifting* means the ability of the body to move, or the mobility of the individual body parts. How important is mobility of the body parts? How important is elasticity or pliability or freedom of the body to move?

When you were a normal, healthy baby, you were completely mobile. Your body could have been rolled into a ball, stretched out like an arrow, twisted right and left like a doorknob, and you would most likely have giggled with glee (see Figure 4).

If you were rolled, twisted, and turned today, however, I doubt that you would gurgle with joy. There would be points of stiffness and strain that more than likely would make you wince. What has happened? Is this normal or not?

The quality of elasticity (mobility, freedom of the body, or pliability) is a characteristic of healthy tissue. The connections that hold our body parts together are yielding and elastic in youth. But time changes this quality.

In the average person, connective tissue *gradually* loses its elastic quality as the person ages, and everyone begins to age the minute he is born. But

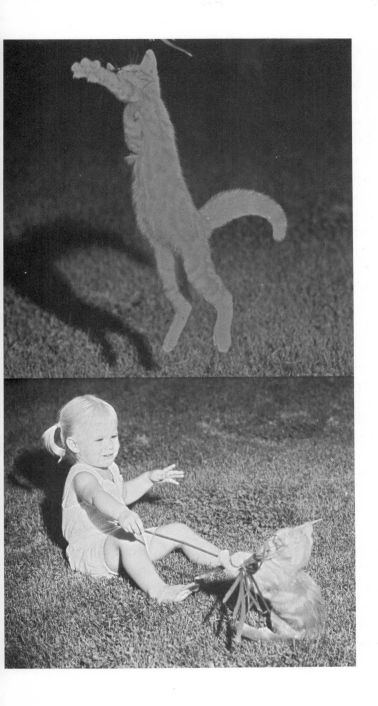

FIGURE 4.
A normal, healthy baby, and pet, are completely mobile. The stretchability of the body bindings is normal in both.

each person's aging process is different. Many factors enter into this, and we will discuss the most important ones that have a bearing on elasticity.

At the age of 20, you should be able to touch the floor with your fingertips, but if you stop short when bending over at the age of 40, beware (see Figure 2). There is no need for this premature shortening. With modern scientific knowledge and techniques, it is quite possible to retain the elasticity of connective tissue that you enjoyed in youth.

A lady from Mexico City was a living example of such youthful elasticity. I met Madame Gaudary through Dr. Arnold Kegel of the University of Southern California Medical School and the Mayo Clinic. When Madame Gaudary came through Los Angeles from Mexico City, she visited the clinic, where I was supervisor of the therapy department.

An attractive woman of grace, poise, and easy movement, she had spent most of her life in Europe and Latin America as a body movement instructor. Among her clients, whose names she guarded closely, were leading government officials and professional personalities. With total ease, Madame Gaudary demonstrated a few movements by reaching down to the floor and, with her legs straight, putting both palms flat on the floor. This she accomplished with very little effort. Then she raised one leg high with the ease of a ballerina, placed it on the desk, and lowered her forehead to her knee.

Impressed by her seemingly limitless flexibility, I commented, "It's wonderful to observe a middle-aged person with the flexibility of a 20-year-old."

Dr. Kegel smiled and said, "I know it is unchivalrous to reveal a lady's age, but in this case, I'm proud to do so. Madame Gaudary is seventy-two!"

We deluged the delightfully young old lady with questions about her physical program. What techniques? What routines? What schedules?

"The answer is simple," she replied. "All my life I've stretched every day. This is fundamental to good posture—also your general health. This is what I teach my clients."

While many decades separate Madame Gaudary from the later astronauts, who were able to stretch while in space, their freedom from stiffness is due to the same thing, the elasticity and yield of their body bindings.

Good muscle development, however desirable for a variety of reasons, won't eliminate tightness of the body bindings in a 72-year-old, and it won't help an astronaut confined in a space capsule.

What about ordinary persons who on occasion get twinges that seem to tell them their joints are stiffening? Is this merely a warning of impending trouble or should this stiffness fill them with fear? Of the thousands of clinic patients who come in for vague distresses, a majority believe that they are hopelessly crippled for life. "I know that I will not walk again," stated one gentleman, whose very painful hip was afflicted with inflammation and tenderness that made walking impossible. After careful medical attention and total restoration of the health of the hip joint, he was put through a stretch program to regain his former range of motion. He walked better than ever when that was accomplished. And, happily, most people's mobility can be restored.

Today's way of living presents additional hazards to the health of our connective tissue. I remember a young married couple—let's call them Mary and Joe—who were victims of an accident that 50 years ago could not have happened to one out of 100,000 persons: whiplash.

Mary and Joe each wore a Thomas collar—a plaster cast around the neck that is a familiar sight in public these days. Usually those who wear them are victims of screeching brakes on the highway.

Waiting for a stop light to change, Joe and Mary had been rear-ended by a huge truck. The truck driver had been listening to a ball game and was oblivious to the red light. In addition to the excruciating pain and stiffness they suffered, they were plagued with double vision and nausea. As a supplement to his complete examination, tests, medication, etc., their medical doctor prescribed heat, massage and very light passive motion until all healing took place. Then a program of stretches was prescribed for complete restoration of range of motion in their necks.

Mary and Joe were both 28 years of age, but in a forward bending position their fingertips stopped far short of the floor (see Figure 2). The range of Mary was like that of a 40-year-old, and Joe's body was even tighter. Yet these were young people. Since she had no interest in active sports, did no walking, and was a housewife who hired a cleaning woman once a week, Mary's exercise was limited entirely to cooking and light dusting. Joe's insurance company desk job kept him seated most of the work day. To be sure, he was dedicated to sports car racing, but this only extended the time he was sitting down since he raced every weekend.

Naturally, a jolt from a truck would unhinge and cause pain in anybody. However, after carefully examining Joe and Mary, it was determined that their high level of joint restriction, stiffness, and overtightness directly corresponded to the unusually extensive tearing they suffered in their necks and shoulders.

The average whiplash injury requires careful medical diagnosis, treatment, and guidance throughout the recovery period. For the reasons spelled out so well in these cases, I advocate a complete stretching program for the whole body *before* such an accident occurs, so that injury is kept to a minimum. It is the observation of many medical doctors and health personnel that the patient who is in good physical shape, with complete range of motion in all body joints before a whiplash injury, has a shorter healing time.

In new buildings today, considerable allowance is made for yield in the event of an earthquake. A new hospital, for example, is built with large spaces between the supporting beams to allow for sway and movement. This is safety planning and implementation. Why not do the same with the human structure? Just a little understanding of the ABC's of your body and the inner power of your structure and its release can make the difference between severe trauma and slight bruising.

This is simple prevention, the kind that is part of every athlete's normal training. No coach would send a man on the football field without preseason training (see Figure 5). For the rest of us, on the freeways and roads, where opportunities for severe in-

FIGURE 5.
Dancers Must Maintain
Complete Body Mobility

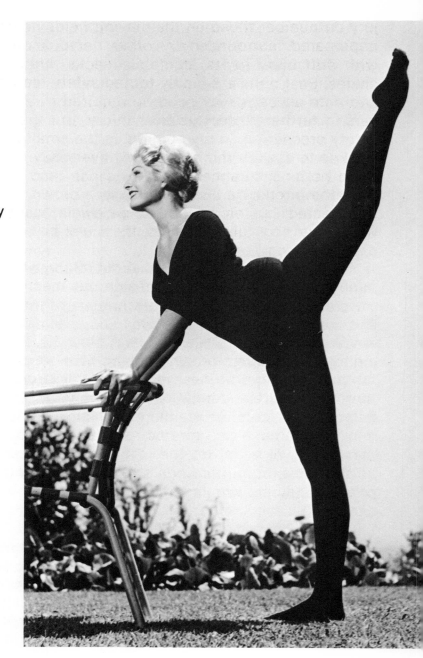

jury outnumber those on the playing field, we drive unprepared, surrounded by other nervous drivers with stiff body joints, immobile necks, hips, and ankles. Seat belts are highly touted safety features, and auto air bags may soon be required in all new cars to further protect us from injury. But the best safety precaution, in my opinion, is the small effort it takes to stretch the entire body every day. There is no better insurance against the pain and injury from the lurch of a bus, a shove in a crowd, or an unexpected fall on a slippery sidewalk, because when your body doesn't yield, there will be a great deal of tearing.

You undoubtedly have heard about rolling with the punches in life; yet this expression has meaning in a literal sense as well. The stretchability of the body and the yield of inner structures will automatically enable the body to give with a hard blow, thus keeping injury to a minimum. In working with poliomyelitis patients on crutches, in addition to stretching their stiff joints and building stronger muscles, we helped them practice yielding in a fall in order to minimize damage to their bodies (see Figure 6). If a person knows he is going to fall down and relaxes to allow the body bindings to stretch as long as possible, tearing will be kept at a minimum, if it occurs at all.

Nature has many lessons for us. Are we paying heed? Why don't animals suffer early joint pain? If you have a dog or cat, some day when you're home all day, count the number of times your pet indulges in a long, luxurious stretch. Animal instincts prompt both canines and felines to stretch at least a dozen

FIGURE 6.
A child, aged three, stricken with polio, could not walk except in water. To keep his muscles active and his connective tissue stretched out to its normal length, he practiced daily in the pool. If you don't use tissue, it will disintegrate.

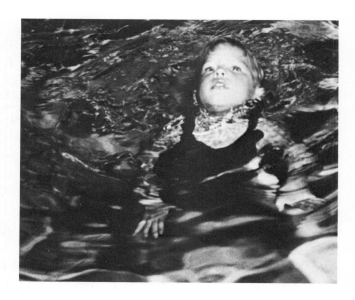

times a day to avoid stiffness. They keep their bodies ready for sudden runs, graceful leaps, dashes into the yard and similar activity. And domestic animals are not the only ones who stretch often. The last time you went to the zoo, you undoubtedly watched the caged lions and tigers pacing, yawning, stretching—constantly stretching, as a matter of fact—to counteract the adverse effects of confinement. Living tissue requires expansion and contraction, and animals are more heedful of nature's demands than most humans.

This built-in instinct to stretch is the basis for the movements you will learn for releasing your body and gaining full mobility. It is fundamental to movement. It can serve you to great advantage if you put it into operation. So once you've learned the stretches, use them!

3 Test Your Self

When Greek culture was at its height, the ideal man not only aspired toward mental perfection; he also disciplined his body. It was believed at the time that noble thoughts could not be housed in a faulty structure.

As we all know, physical and emotional strains in modern living are not decreasing, and these must be released in a healthy manner. Can we help ourselves? What must we learn in order to cope with this modern dilemma?

Do not be incredulous when I say that with very little time, effort, and a minimum amount of skill, you can overcome the threat of having a faulty structure house your mental capabilities. The most easily achievable perfection can be the physical, and age is not a factor. Your years don't determine a youthful appearance or physical and mental health. Rather, flexibility—or the lack of it—gives the impression of one's age. A relaxed, painfree way of moving and a well-functioning body will make you look young; stiff movements suggest aging. Yet tight joints can easily be loosened. How?

Before you institute a program of elongation of the body bindings, you must learn to test the range of motion of your body segments. Where is it adequate? Where is it faulty? Is full mobility present, and at what points is it incomplete?

Let us start at the top—the head and neck. At the base of the skull, there is a very thick band of bindings and we will test the mobility of these first. If you have completely normal range of motion in the neck region, you will be able to roll your head forward, sideways, and backward with ease, and in order to have this range of motion, you must be able to move your head 90 degrees to each side (see Test 1, Figure 7).

If they are entirely free and mobile, the body bindings will permit your head to turn to either the right or the left with ease and comfort. If they are stiff and inflexible, they will stop your head from making a complete 90-degree turn. If the shortening of these neck bindings continues for several years, it can cause enough discomfort to send a person in pursuit of medical care.

Do not be surprised to find that you are not able to bring your chin all the way over the tip of your shoulder. Many people cannot. One case in particular comes to mind.

A writer for motion picture and television studios complained bitterly of constant headaches. "You have got to help me. I can't continue on medication forever, but the minute I don't take anything I have an insufferable headache. I have got to get rid of this and find another way to get relief."

We sat him in a chair, anchored his arms at the side, and hooked his feet around the legs of the chair. In this position, I gently moved his chin to the right, and before I had turned it even 45 degrees he screamed with pain. Without assistance he could hardly turn his head at all without feeling intense pull and strain at the back of his neck and up over his scalp almost to his eyebrows. Since he was well aware of the pain and stiffness, over the years he had prescribed a variety of pills for himself to get rid of headaches. But one simple test would have revealed to him the gradual deterioration of his neck bindings and their inability to yield because they had grown so short. I asked the writer if he had ever

FIGURE 7.
Test 1: Neck Mobility
Normal range in the neck region permits you to turn your head to each side at a 90-degree angle to your shoulders and hips, which are well anchored to the chair.

To test this range, sit in a straight-back chair with your hips well back and your shoulders touching the back of the chair. Both arms should hang close to the sides of your body, and you should grasp the seat near the rear legs of the chair. In this position, turn your head to the side as far as possible until your chin is directly over the tip of your shoulder. You should then turn your head to the opposite side until your chin is aligned with the tip of your shoulder.

Are you entirely comfortable when your head is turned all the way? Again, with a completely free neck, you should be able to turn your head in either direction, right or left, and bring your chin around a full 90 degrees.

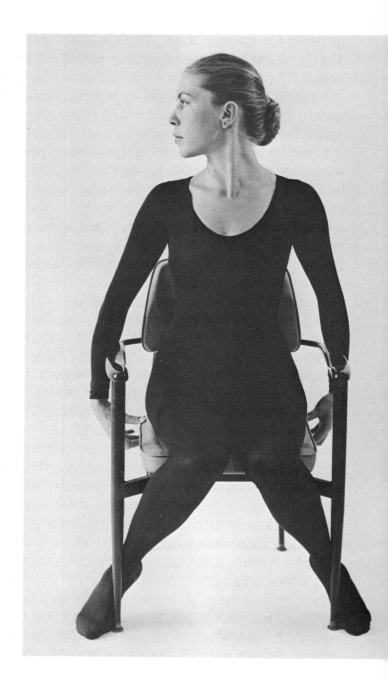

38

gone in for sports or any physical activities, and he shook his head. "I just want to get rid of these headaches."

"You don't have to learn a sport to do that," I replied, "but you probably have to move to get moving again."

I had to prepare him for a movement program that would promote a gradual but steady loosening of his neck bindings to get them back to or at least close to their original lengths. It took much coaxing, explaining, daily discipline, and help to restore comfortable neck movements to this person. His therapy had to undo 20 years of neglect, inactivity, abuse, and almost complete immobility. The medical clinics are full of such people.

Tight necks are not confined to writers. They are an occupational hazard for everyone who spends many hours hunched over, whether at a desk, ironing board, sewing machine, or whatever. If the position is not counteracted with stretch movements, the body's original range of motion is diminished. But not forever; fortunately it is correctable, although the longer one waits, the harder it is to accomplish. Tissue yields, as long as it is alive. Astounding as it may seem, persons well along in years —in their sixties and seventies—have successfully elongated their body bindings. Even many of them can hardly believe it, but it happens. They prove it to themselves, and so will you, provided you give stretching a fair try.

A particularly stubborn stiff neck case was that of Mr. L, an executive in his sixties. He had a long history of diabetes, which was controlled by daily insulin injections. He was plagued by repeated morning headaches, for which he was given power-ful medication. These complicated his insulin in-take. His orthopedic specialist suggested that since diabetes was primarily a glandular imbalance and since such chemical imbalances affect connective tissue and shorten it, this shortening must have been aggravating his neck ligaments. Before we set out to test the range of motion in the neck region, we observed two other factors that might also have been contributing to the shortening. Mr. L's tall, rigid posture bespoke a tension that seemed to be centered in his neck. An executive of great impor-tance who did a great deal of reading, writing, and administrative work at his desk, he felt obliged to maintain an erect and rigid posture that emanated efficiency and authority—a position for which his neck bindings were paying dearly. Suffice it to say that a regimen of heat, passive stretches, and man-ipulations was performed on the patient before he arrived at a point where he could carry on neck stretching movements by himself to achieve com-plete neck mobility and relief from a great deal of discomfort.

Another case that illustrates the need for checking the range of motion in the upper back was that of Danny, a photographer. He was stricken with a sharp pain in his chest while shooting several beach lay-outs in Santa Monica. Beginning in his left shoulder, the pain was so sharp and traveled so fast over his shoulder and down his arm that he was certain he was having a heart attack.

He walked slowly to his car and drove quickly to his doctor's office. After checking out his heart for three hours, the doctor informed Danny that his heart was normal and that there was no sign of cardiac deficiency.

But upper spine and neck X-rays showed that Danny had some minor arthritis, not uncommon at the age of 50. His physician diagnosed the chest pains as coming from shortened ligaments in his neck and upper spine, aggravated by fatigue caused by carrying too much heavy photographic equipment. He also stated that the morning fog at the beach did not agree with Danny's body bindings, since sudden exposure to cold can cause further contractions of tissue already shortened at the joints, creating very sharp pain.

For Danny, a long overdue program of neck and shoulder stretches was begun to give him relief. Had he gone the prevention route and stretched regularly over the years, the increased circulation would have helped to keep the arthritic processes at a minimum, if they occurred at all, and the pliability of his upper back would have been maintained at the normal range. He showed me the leg kicks he performed on his back that had been his former conditioning program; these exercises did absolutely nothing for his range of motion at any point.

If you have complete range of motion in your upper spine, you should be able to perform Test 2 (see Figure 8) without any pull or strain at any point. The motion should be comfortable, and only you can tell how it feels. If it is not comfortable, you will have to elongate your body bindings in this area, but fortunately, this can be done very easily. Whether the tightness is minimal or severe, it can be alleviated.

The third and last test evaluates the range of motion in all areas of the lower part of the body (see Figure 9, Test 3). It is trouble in this portion of the body that sends most people to the medical clinics with aches and pains after many years of neglect and immobility. With body stretching as a preventive measure, thousands of individuals can delay the deterioration that comes with middle and old age. Physical decline is not inevitable if you are willing to help yourself, as many people, some famous and some not so famous, have demonstrated. King Gustav of Sweden played tennis at 85 years of age. May Sutton, two-time Wimbledon champion, won tennis tournaments at 85 years of age. Mrs. Carrie Jones, age 73, a not-so-famous example, gardens daily, bending and twisting as if she were 40 years of age without any discomfort whatsoever.

Many college students fail the third test of mobility, even athletic male students, because their sports emphasize lower body strength at the expense of body range and joint loosening. A stretch program where it is needed, however, corrects the tightness in a relatively short time. Correction at this stage is extremely simple; young body bindings are still very elastic and can yield easily, if put into the stretching position. Neglect is what we must avoid if we want safety, comfort, and freedom in our later years.

If you want to check your overall body mobility again, you can test the flexibility of all posterior bindings, not just the separate segments as in Tests 1, 2, and 3. The posterior bindings are continuous and are especially thickened in their attachments at the base of the neck, bottom of the spine, and at the back of the heels (see Figure 11). To test the bindings, see Figure 12. If you checked out stiffly in Test 3, you will feel very tight cords at the sides of your knees as you bend forward. They will feel like steel cables if they are very tight, and they are why your fingers cannot touch the floor when you bend forward with your knees straight. Your connective tissue just won't let you extend all the way down. It holds you like a clamp or rope that won't give. But again, this can be changed!

So now you see that even though a certain amount of body binding shortening goes with aging, you can nevertheless test for those parts that have shortened too much, determining not only your general body flexibility, but picking out the real trouble spots that need special emphasis in the lengthening process. With that knowledge, you need only to learn the next step: how to correct your tightness.

Put your own power to work to achieve a better physical structure. And what could be better than using the incredible mechanism that nature gave to us? As Julian Huxley, the famous biologist, so aptly stated, "Man has not yet begun to recognize the phenomenon of his physical structure."

FIGURE 8.
Test 2: Upper Trunk Mobility

To test the range in your upper back, sit in a straight-back chair. Keep your hips well back and hook your feet around the front legs of the chair. Turn your shoulders to the right and "help" the turn by "climbing" around the chair with your arms. You should be able to turn the upper part of your body a full 90 degrees while your hips remain stationary. Repeat to the left. When you force your shoulders to the complete 90-degree turn, do you feel a pull at the back of your shoulders? At your spine? At your ribs? Or is this position perfectly comfortable and easy to hold?

FIGURE 9.
Test 3

Sit with one leg resting on a table or support of some kind, at a right angle to your hips. In this position, keep your toes pointing upward. Do you feel any pull at your hip? At your knee? At your ankle? Or is this position perfectly comfortable to your legs and the rest of your body?

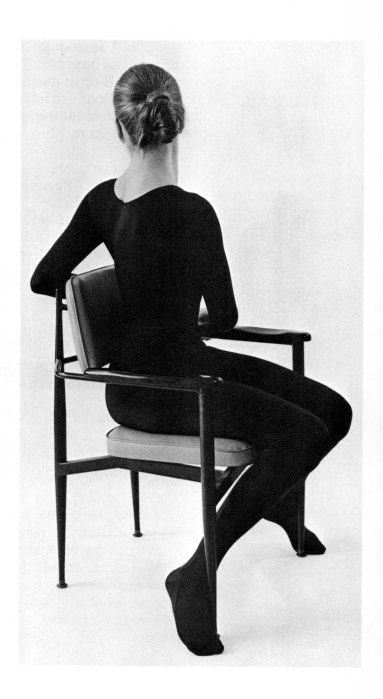

44

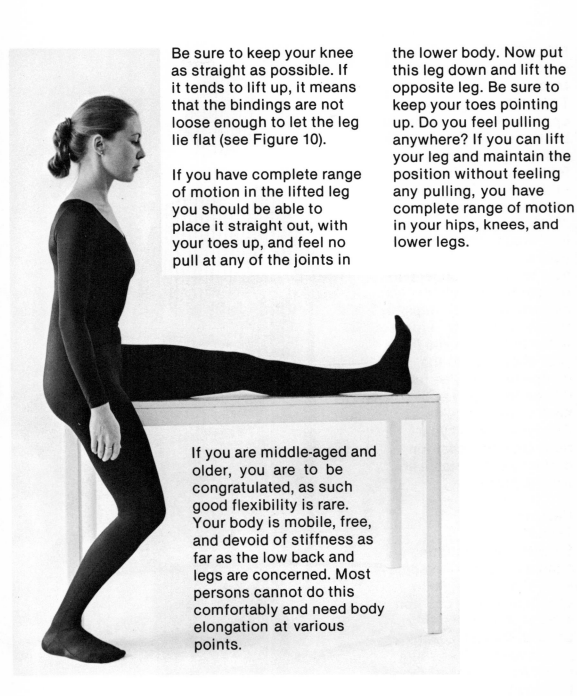

Be sure to keep your knee as straight as possible. If it tends to lift up, it means that the bindings are not loose enough to let the leg lie flat (see Figure 10).

If you have complete range of motion in the lifted leg you should be able to place it straight out, with your toes up, and feel no pull at any of the joints in the lower body. Now put this leg down and lift the opposite leg. Be sure to keep your toes pointing up. Do you feel pulling anywhere? If you can lift your leg and maintain the position without feeling any pulling, you have complete range of motion in your hips, knees, and lower legs.

If you are middle-aged and older, you are to be congratulated, as such good flexibility is rare. Your body is mobile, free, and devoid of stiffness as far as the low back and legs are concerned. Most persons cannot do this comfortably and need body elongation at various points.

FIGURE 10.
The male student's legs
are held bent at the knee
because of overshortening
in his hip and leg bindings.
In a simple sitting position,
with arms held overhead,
his body bindings do not
allow his leg to lie straight.
Notice the difference in
the female partner, whose
leg lies fairly flat, with a
smaller space under the
knee. Her longer bindings
allow this.

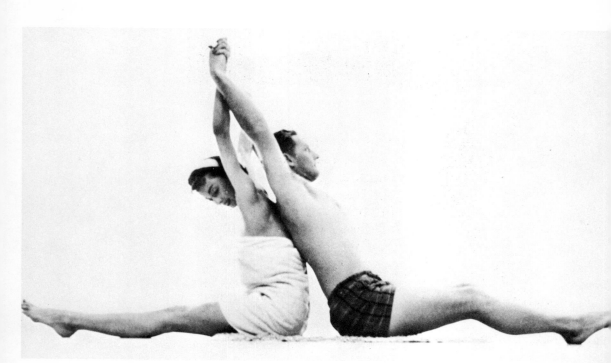

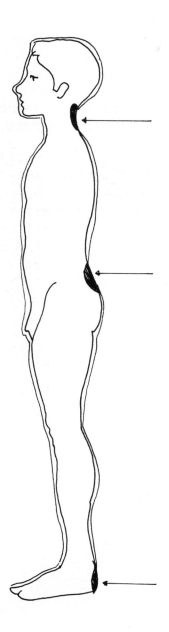

FIGURE 11.
Body bindings (ligaments) are continuous. They are particularly thick at the base of the skull, base of the spine, and the heel.

47

FIGURE 12.
Total Body Flexibility
Standing with your feet together and knees straight, lower your trunk to the floor, allowing your arms to hang loosely. Try to touch the floor with your fingertips. Keep your knees straight throughout. Come up slowly. Relax.

In early adult life—up to 35 years of age—one should be able to touch or come close to the floor with the fingertips. Later, the body shortens and becomes less elastic, so that the fingertips may not readily reach the floor but stop about five inches away (see Figure 2). If this much stiffness is present at 30, it must be corrected. It can be done easily; with daily practice the fingers will soon reach the floor.

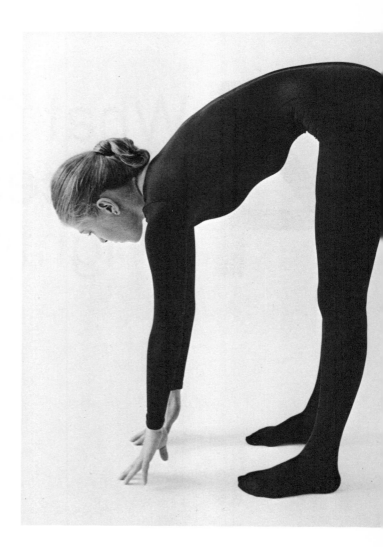

4 What Causes Excessive Tightness?

Why Tight?

Before we begin the elongation program for short-ened bindings, we need to examine the various complaints associated with body stiffness. What causes excessive shortening? We have mentioned the factor of aging. Are there other causes? And if so, what are they, and are they avoidable?

The program of stretching is not merely another set of exercises or a design to keep moving. Many reliable authorities tell people that they should keep moving in order to prevent the loss of their ability to move, and in this space age that is correct, but it is not quite enough.

What joy is there in life if one reaches middle age and has kinks, disturbances, and body discomfort that prevent participation in activities and preclude a happy disposition? Nearly everyone at some time or another has had a toothache. Although it is cen-tered in only an extremely small area of the body, that pain can cause a feeling of sickness all over the body that makes life pretty miserable while it lasts.

And so it is with other areas of the body that send off distress signals. These messages to us can be ignored, can be overstressed, or can be met with corrective measures. You can take your choice.

Exercise is a scientific tool; each conditioning technique achieves a different purpose. One can jog to increase fitness of the heart and blood vessels of the body; and large firm muscles, for increased strength, are built through resistive exercises.

Increased vitality and increased muscle strength are very important in certain lifestyles, activities, and pursuits (see Figure 13); however, they don't contribute to the range of motion in movement. You

50

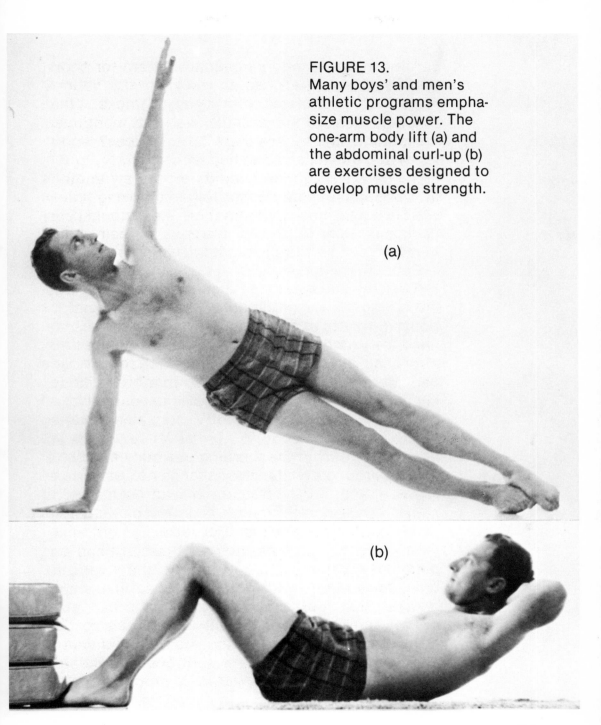

FIGURE 13.
Many boys' and men's athletic programs emphasize muscle power. The one-arm body lift (a) and the abdominal curl-up (b) are exercises designed to develop muscle strength.

(a)

(b)

Why Tight?

can jog from here to Timbuktu and never correct bothersome low back pain caused by overtight lower back bindings. In fact, you may aggravate that condition because of the jarring and bouncing. You can build impressive biceps and Mr. Universe chest contours and still experience headaches and scalp tension from overstiff neck bindings. As a matter of fact, you most likely *will* suffer this stiffness unless you have paid particular attention to elongating your neck and upper trunk muscles to counteract the effects of your overdeveloped musculature.

Some very simple observations can clue you in as to whether you need a stretch program, even without taking the three tests checking each part of the body. If it hurts to get up and down from a chair, you need to stretch. If you are uncomfortable, especially after long periods of sitting, you are most likely a candidate for elongation. If you reach for the top shelf and can't quite make it because your neck and shoulders are stiff, you should consider restoring that part of your body to normal range. If you are unbearably stiff in the morning but feel easier after moving around a while; if your hands do not close all the way; and, finally, if your neck turns are getting shorter and shorter, you should seriously contemplate changing all that (see Figure 14).

Reshaping programs, cosmetic alterations, and diets are popular paths to follow in the search for the elusive fountain of youth. You need only go on a guided travel tour to observe those who look great at first, but whose bodies wilt disastrously as they que in long lines, walk on cobbles for any distance, and climb uphill. Their tight, stiff bodies impolitely remind them of deterioration way beyond normal for their years, and their sagging, fatigued facial muscles add on the age they have striven so hard to hide. In a medical clinic program, where one sees many people suffering from severe pain, it is gratifying to see people look 10 years younger when the pain in their joints is alleviated and the original, youthful function of motion is restored.

You yourself have the power to make the change toward a youthful appearance and, above all, better health. Just reestablish your original body range.

Let us get better acquainted with the body bindings, which clearly have greater significance than most people think. First, do not think that your body bindings are fragile and easily torn. This is not true. Connective tissue is extremely tough, composed of multiple layers of cells interwoven into extremely resilient bands at the points of attachment to bone, and this is absolutely necessary, because it takes a great deal of jarring and jolting in ordinary walking, standing, or sitting. Its function is a long, steady one. Small wonder that it "complains" occasionally and may even snap angrily into a tight, unyielding encasement, letting us know that it has had enough.

Connective bindings, or ligaments, have the quality of contractility as well as elasticity. The contractility persists throughout life, but elasticity changes; it decreases with age. The degree differs with each person, but in general it lessens very gradually unless it is badly abused. The contractile quality of the connective tissue supersedes all other qualities; in other words, the tissue tends to contract. The attachments that bind the tissue to the bone have especially thick segments (knee joint, heel cord, etc.), and tend to shorten after a period of

FIGURE 14.
Range of motion from the
hips down is restricted in
the male. He cannot
straighten his leg comfortable

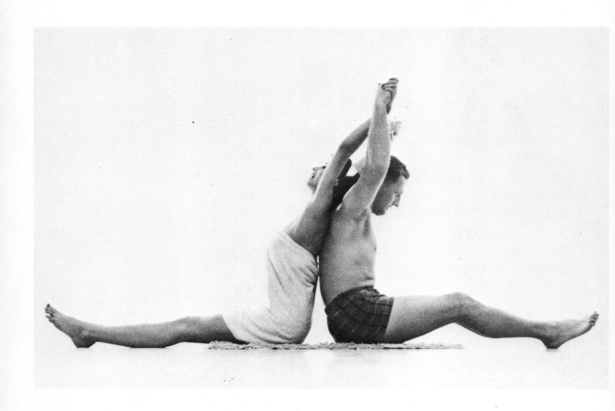

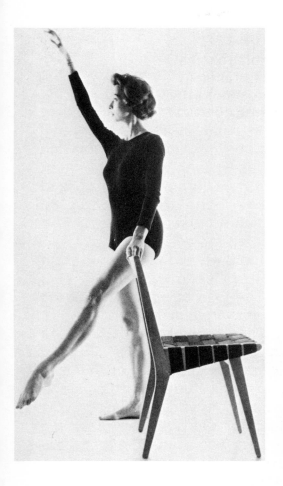

An ankle that has complete range of movement can elongate to a straight line and come up to a 90-degree angle

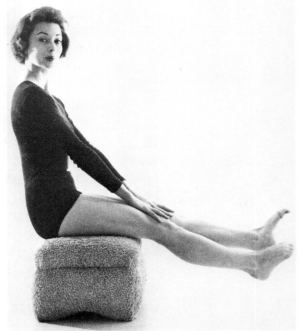

Why Tight?

heavy activity followed by a period of inactivity. This property is well demonstrated in athletes—especially high hurdlers, high jumpers or vaulters—who must undergo intensive training, extensive stretching, and long limbering-up periods after a spell of inactivity before the season starts. The ordinary person experiences this to a certain extent after curling into a ball at night while sleeping; usually he must stretch out the next morning upon getting up and walking around. Performers who are cooped up on tour between performances must warm up before they go on stage, loosening the body bindings.

So the tendency for the body bindings to shorten remains, and the quality of elasticity does not. This is an important point. The loss of elasticity should be gradual and easy, not severe and marked.

What causes excessive shortening? What are the abuses that contribute to the contractility?

One of the most common causes of shortening of the ligaments is poor posture. Students, office workers, cashiers, and anyone else who sits a good part of the time in his occupation has a tendency to drop his head and neck forward. The spine then compensates for this position and goes into a round back configuration. When the tissues are held in this posture over many years, the bindings adapt to it; in other words, they remain fixed in a shortened position. When the person wishes to stretch his neck, shoulders, and upper spine, he is literally held in the forward-curved position if he has practiced faulty body mechanics for many years. Yet he is only aware that it does not feel comfortable to straighten up; it not only hurts but it feels odd. He is so used to the forward-curved position of his neck and back that he has the wrong impression that it is normal. Only when neck and shoulder pains begin, when excessive tightening has taken over, is the person aware that something is wrong. Quite often in such cases the person cannot lie flat on his back on the floor or exercise mat to perform some movements. His neck and shoulders will not flatten to the floor, and he has to use pillows. In old age these persons are the ones who have to be propped up in bed with many pillows to support the head and neck and to fill in the space between their backs and the back of the bed. The bindings will no longer yield to hold the spine and neck in a straight position, which will enable them to sit against the back of the bed.

A famous celebrity, an internationally known violinist, had a forward-fixed head. When he was referred for neck and shoulder mobilization, he could not lie on his back without the support of two pillows. His head would not lie flat because of excessive tissue shortening. At 72 years of age it is not so simple to elongate body attachments that have been held shortened for 50 years. Fortunately, however, they can yield somewhat even at that late date.

Another common source of shortening are strains and sprains. Strains that tear the little fibers in the connective tissue are an all-too-common experience. There may be intense pain at the moment of the strain, as in lifting a heavy object or a sudden twist in attempting to regain balance in a fall. But the pain passes quickly and the individual continues his chores. The next day, however, is another story. "I could hardly get out of bed," one badminton player reported after having twisted the lower part of his back in a fall during a game. "It did not hurt me at the time of the fall. I just knew that I had twisted a bit at the hip trying to regain my balance." The next morning, however, this player could not move without feeling sharp pains at both sides low in his back. He could not bend, twist, or move without severe pain, and his back was stiff as a board at the lower end. He had to roll out of bed. The muscle spasm that he was feeling was nature's way of supporting the fibers that were torn when he twisted. One week later, this player was completely out of pain. He had kept moving even though there was pain, and he broke the vicious cycle of joint protection and complete immobility that would only have caused greater stiffness.

Whenever an injury of this type takes place, continued stretches are indicated to keep scars at a minimum in size. Scar tissue is made up of white fibers that are tough and inelastic. When there is stress upon such tissue, the adjacent nerve pathways can be greatly irritated and transmit pain to the brain. To bring in more circulation and vascularize this area is highly desirable for future body comfort, and this can be accomplished through stretching. Very often persons report injuries or falls in their youth. After many years they feel irritation at the joint concerned and wonder about the problem. When reminded that there may once have been tearing at the joint, they become aware that they never corrected the tightness or scarring that "puckered" for years and eventually interfered with range of motion.

The quality of scarring tissue to pucker is the reason one is advised to massage ointments and creams into visible scars on the skin. This keeps them vascularized, pliable, and elongated. The only way one can achieve the same results with nonvisible scars, namely those in the soft inner tissues of the body, is to stretch. Stretching brings accelerated circulation and general cell nourishment to the scarred area and helps prevent puckering.

Another contributor to excessive shortening is traceable to the glandular system. Gland changes and instabilities affect the quality of connective tissue but must be determined by a medical authority. One of the common gland-related fluctuations, however, is the menstrual cycle, in which the estrogen level in women is lowered during monthly periods. The hyperirritability of the whole pelvic region at this time and the subsequent contracting of the connective tissue can cause great discomfort and is a condition that schoolteachers have had to contend with in dealing with adolescent girls. In former decades students experiencing such discomfort were sent to rest periods to become wholly inactive and supposedly release the tension that was causing the pain. Now, however, we not only do not advise students to rest and abstain from movement, we prescribe very special stretches and movements to counteract the overshortening and hence relieve that nerve irritation that is at the root of the problem.

Certain diseases and conditions such as arthritis, malaria, influenza, and paretic muscles, can also bring about excessive shortening of the body bindings. Arthritis is one of the most notorious cripplers affecting the body bindings. It does not rank among the top three killer diseases, but as a source of chronic pain and stiffness, it dominates the scene. In reviewing all the arthritis cases that I have worked with, I recalled that the overwhelming majority of patients were Caucasian. There were few blacks, Latins, or American Indians. I wrote to a friend, Paula Crain, who was a Seminole Indian in Oklahoma and an education specialist for the Seminole and Creek Indians at Wewoka, Oklahoma. As a scholar of Indian folklore and medicine, perhaps she could offer some clue or insight into connective tissue damage caused by arthritis.

She wrote back: "Diseases such as muscular or joint ailments are rare among these tribes. Outdoor life accounts for hardiness and immunizes them against such complaints as joint stiffness. As for paralysis, not a single case of this most dreaded disease, so prevalent among other races, ever occurred among the older Indians—no curvature of spine, crooked limbs, or body deformities [those due to faulty body mechanics such as round backs, sway backs, locked knees, etc.]. These seem not to have affected these people. Getting away from the simple life of their ancestors has had a tendency to shorten the life span of this once-hardy race, however, since adopting the mode of modern living. To those who know and admire the modest life of the true American, it is with much regret and sadness that we witness the diminishing of a once-noble race."

Another common occurrence causing excessive tightening, and one that is experienced by many persons, is a sudden drastic temperature change.

"We went for a beautiful ride last night, in the warm, balmy breeze, but when we hit the ocean there was a considerable fog."

"Was your car window open at the time?"

"Oh yes. The cooling breeze felt good after all that heat."

To state that the good feeling dissolved into a stiff, aching neck the next morning would be an understatement. The pain this person had was intolerable. Like many others, he was feeling the results of overshortening caused by sudden temperature change. The bodies of such people are sensitive and react to any temperature drop that is sudden or severe. A stretch program, performed daily, keeps the overshortening to a minimum and provides a palliative procedure when the body reacts. Dropping your chin to your chest, rolling your head in a complete circle, and turning your chin to the side over your shoulder—all done daily under a hot shower— can keep your neck attachments at a normal length.

Even if your body is not overly sensitive to temperature change, this daily routine is advisable to counteract the effects of the sedentary nature of modern living. The Guatemalan women who daily carry their wash on their heads to the town fountains do not need neck mobilization and posture training. Their baskets would fall if they had drooping heads and shoulders, so they have stretched their necks tall since youth. Our necks, on the other hand, need stretching to compensate for the effects of stooping over the washing machine and the desk calculator.

To repeat, the main causes of overshortened body bindings are habitual poor posture, excessive strains and tears, emotional stress, glandular deficiencies of various sorts (medically determined), sudden temperature changes, and various diseases. Excessive shortening can produce some very com-

Why Tight?

mon symptoms that are interpreted as headaches, back aches, leg pains, and foot pains, and these symptoms can be eliminated through a stretch program. More important, however, they can be prevented by stretches that you alone can do. This is known as *delayed deterioration.* Even though it is impossible to turn the clock back to simpler times, we can prevent premature erosion of our body parts, and the details of such prevention are worth a hard look.

Stretches are simple, uncomplicated, easy to learn. They are goal oriented, and progress toward that goal can be measured objectively. They provide a means to become healthier while we grow older! One of the best contributions we can make to our later years is to prepare for the best possible health in our early and middle years. Opportunities in old age are 100 percent dependent upon good health, and help toward that good health begins in the next chapter.

5 Stay Loose- 3 Stretches That Can Change Your Life

Stay
Loose

One of the best and most important resolutions you can make for your future health is a daily program of stretching. The relaxation you derive from limbering up with only three basic stretches not only will cut down on tension and fatigue but will enable you to move with an ease and comfort that you haven't felt for years.

Since the stretches advocated in this book are essentially preventive measures, it is assumed that those participating are still in a nondeteriorated state as far as general health is concerned. For most people the stretches are simple movements that can be performed without medical supervision. If a person has had an illness, accident, or injury, however, medical consent should be obtained. When orthopedists warn a patient that he should never bend forward with his knees straight, for example, they have a very good medical reason for this advice. Certain injuries or disease processes can be aggravated by this position. This book is not directed to such people; they need medical therapists to guide them through corrective movements.

The majority of people still have healthy structures, however, and motion and activity are absolutely necessary to maintain that health. Stretches are an excellent means toward that goal.

To be truly effective, you should do the three basic stretches in a simple routine, and you must do them correctly if you wish to achieve the scientific result for which they are designed. It takes just a little learning and not too great an effort.

You will start to loosen the neck and upper torso first and then work down to the lower back, knees, and lower legs. In this manner you will loosen the entire torso from head to toe and will reflect this looseness in all your movements. Who can dispute the gracefulness of the cat or dog who starts stretching at the front and gracefully extends that stretch to the rear section until its entire body is extended in readiness for smooth, sudden movement? Humans have the same capacity and similar equipment to do it.

The following simple rules will help you get the very best results.

Do your stretches a specific number of times. Set your routine at 3, 5, 10, or whatever. Each person will be different. If you feel a pull, do not stop. It will disappear the minute you release your stretch. The greater the pull you feel, the more you need the stretch, because it means the connections are tight.

Surrender the body part you are stretching; that is, make it yield. Have the feeling that you are letting go completely. When you are working on the neck, for example, concentrate on that one section and "speak" to it. Say "Let go," and surrender completely to the turn, going as far as possible. When you hit a block of resistance, go a little bit farther even if you feel a pull. This is the sign of a very successful stretch and one that you ultimately will be able to do without any stress pulls when that part of your body is entirely freed from restriction.

Do your stretches daily. It will take less than five minutes for three stretches to loosen your entire torso. Tissues will give, but to make them yield is a gradual process, and consequently the lengthening will take time. A daily pull at the crucial areas will accomplish the lengthening for you. Frequent short intervals of stretching (some persons do it twice a day) will help you toward flexibility better than long-er, less frequent periods. The stretching is aimed at increasing the range of motion of body parts, not endurance, so the short periods can easily accom-plish the goal. Daily stretching can keep body stiff-ening and tightening at a minimum. It is a matter of personal discipline to incorporate this health rou-tine into your daily schedule.

Each of the three stretches has been applied over many years of practice and administered to young people as well as middle-aged and older. Success can be achieved at any age.

In Test 3 you learned how close your forehead could come to your knee when you have one leg slightly elevated. If the distance was great, you need elongation. In Stretch 3 you can determine where the greatest point of tightness is located. If you feel the pull in your hips only as you bend forward, that is the principal trouble spot and it is not too severe, just slight. If the pull extends further down to the sides of your knee, however, the tightness in your hips is more than slight. And if you feel the pain all the way down to the back of your lower leg and an-kle, there is marked tightness of the bindings.

Since no two bodies are alike and since the hu-man structure allows for great variety of movement, some slightly altered positions are suggested for those who find sitting on the floor difficult. The very same areas are stretched, but you sit in a chair in-stead of on the floor.

For healthy structures, then, motion and activity are essential. And, as you will discover after doing them, the three basic stretches are an excellent means toward that goal.

FIGURE 15.
Stretch 1
To loosen the side attachments of the neck and upper shoulders, sit on the floor with your legs crossed tailor fashion in order to lock your hips so they won't move. Place your chin in your right palm.

Turn your neck as far to the right as possible. When you cannot go any farther, force your chin gently but firmly a little bit farther. Then release slowly and carefully.

Start with three stretches to the right and then three to the left. Increase the number of stretches weekly so that a gradual loosening can take place. To remove any soreness, take a very hot shower particularly directed to the neck.

Those whose movement is very restricted can do this neck stretch with their backs to the wall. Pin your shoulders and hips firmly to the wall; you can then judge how far away your chin is from the wall. When you can touch the wall comfortably with your chin, you are completely free of restriction.

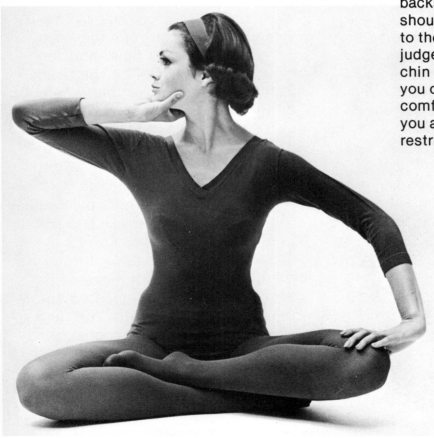

FIGURE 16.

Stretch 2

To loosen your shoulders and upper back, sit on the floor, tailor fashion. Take a mop handle, stick, or large rubber band and place it behind your shoulders. Hold the ends, keeping your arms straight. Slowly twist your trunk as far to the right as possible, until you feel a pull. Then return front and twist to the left. You should do 3 twists to each side daily.

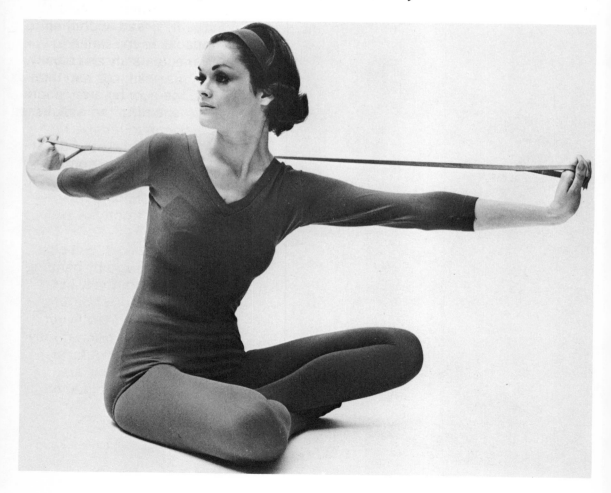

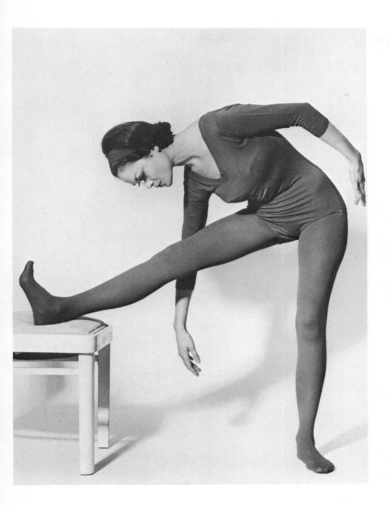

FIGURE 17.
Stretch 3
To loosen your lower back, knees, and leg bindings down to the heel cord, place your right leg on a chair whose seat is approximately at the level of your knee. Bend loosely from the waist, lowering your forehead and trying to touch it to your knee.
Come up easily and slowly. Do this stretch three times and then change to the left leg, repeating three times.

After three weeks your forehead should come down farther. If it does not, you are not doing this stretch correctly.

You might double-check your technique by bending forward from the waist with your legs straight and trying to touch your fingers to the floor. If they are coming down farther than before, you are elongating the bindings successfully.

FIGURE 18.
Stretch 1: Variation
The important thing to remember in doing the neck stretch in a chair is to hook your feet around the legs of the chair. When you stretch any part, you have to move against a fixed point, and by hooking your feet, the hips remain stationary. In addition, the arm you are not using in the stretch should hold onto the chair so that your shoulders also remain stationary.

The movement of your head and neck remains the same, however, as if you were sitting. Place your chin in your palm and turn your head to the side; gently push your chin a little farther to complete the turn. Stretch three times to each side.

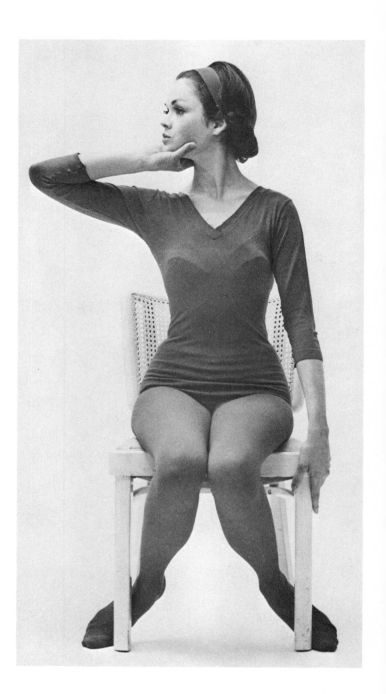

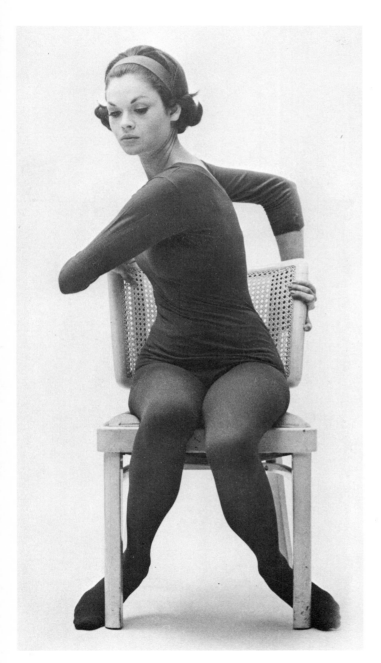

FIGURE 19.
Stretch 2: Variation
To stretch your upper back and shoulders while you are sitting in a chair, hook your feet around the legs of the chair. With your arms, "climb" around the back of the chair until your shoulders are at a 90-degree angle to your hips. Twist as far as possible and give a decided pull. Release slowly. Stretch 3 times to each side.

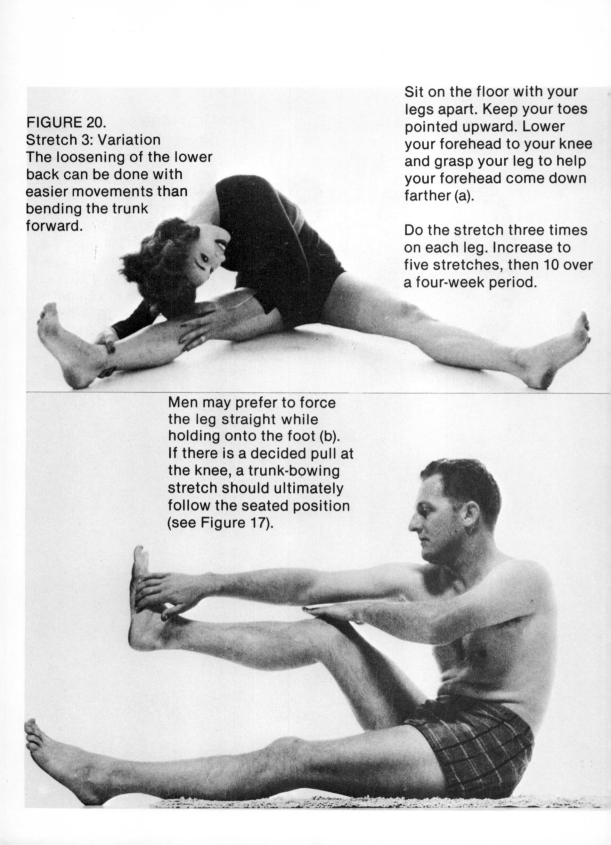

FIGURE 20.
Stretch 3: Variation
The loosening of the lower back can be done with easier movements than bending the trunk forward.

Sit on the floor with your legs apart. Keep your toes pointed upward. Lower your forehead to your knee and grasp your leg to help your forehead come down farther (a).

Do the stretch three times on each leg. Increase to five stretches, then 10 over a four-week period.

Men may prefer to force the leg straight while holding onto the foot (b). If there is a decided pull at the knee, a trunk-bowing stretch should ultimately follow the seated position (see Figure 17).

6 Stretch While You Rest

While
You
Rest

For those of you who do not really enjoy exercising or those who wish a very mild, untaxing routine, the following stretches are meant for you. You can do them while you are relaxing on the patio, at the poolside, or in bed before you get up for the day, while you lounge, sun, or half doze. What could be simpler than stretching while you are resting!

You may wonder what value there is in this, since very little energy is expended while you are resting. Oxygen intake is not increased greatly as in jogging, nor are muscle power, endurance, or coordination developed as in other fitness programs. The effectiveness of stretching has very little to do with energy output. Its objective is to elongate the body bindings. This can be done with little effort, with moderate effort, or very actively, depending on the routine that you prefer.

The resting routine is recommended for the not-so-active individuals—those middle-aged or older or individuals recuperating from a physical incapacity of long standing. These persons and many others can benefit from energy-saving movements. To engage in a meaningful exercise program that aims at minimal exertion but has great importance for the body is not easy to come by. The techniques are not borrowed from Eastern philosophies nor do they require positions foreign to Western culture. They call upon natural instincts in all of us—namely the need to stretch.

To put a natural instinct into operation does not call for medical supervision. These simple resting routines can be done by nearly everyone, without any medical consultation, and this applies to all ages and both sexes. There is, however, one very important exception. If you have had a history of illness, injury, or any pathology whatsoever, medical consent is desirable. A doctor will surely advise against the stretches if there is any swelling, redness, or soreness. Admittedly, exercise is often prescribed to treat arthritis, but it is done under medical supervision and by a trained therapist. That supervision is essential when pathology is present or has been in the recent past.

These stretches are designed to prevent body deterioration. They promote and maintain good body function and comfortable motion. The best test of the effectiveness of your stretches is whether you feel better; function better; and reach, turn, twist, and move better. You can judge the results yourself.

It has been stated by many that Americans are the most undisciplined people in the world. Sister Kenny of Australia, the polio fighter, observed, "Leave it to the Americans to invent a machine to take the place of any physical labor."

The industrial genius of our people has plunged us into a technocratic civilization, but we must not let body function succumb to it. Mechanization of body functions could destroy the freedom and mobility of our youthful elasticity. Biologically we still have movable body parts and the maintenance of that movability is what is at stake. The lure of having it moved for us versus the physiological need to move the part ourselves is the challenge I am referring to. Therein lies our power: to stay loose we have to keep moving; to stay young we have to stretch.

As in the three basic stretches discussed in Chapter 5, the key to a good stretch while resting is the concept of surrendering the part being stretched. Think of a water pump. When a squeeze is put on it, it empties. When it is released, it slowly fills up again. A muscle with constant contraction (squeeze) does not get a chance to refill completely. But upon release, blood flows through to the tiniest capillary, nourishing the cells with a fresh oxygen supply. So releasing or surrendering is the key to furnishing the cells with nourishment. This affects the overall health of the body; therefore a great emphasis should be placed upon relaxation or release of the body part during and after a stretch.

If you are now ready for your stretches, lie on your back. Your hips should be higher than your head and your knees higher than your hips (see Figure 21). Your spine is straight and your organs in proper place. Count to 100. Then "speak" to your body and say, "Let go; let go." Then do the stretch shown in Figure 22. After 10 stretches for each side, take three deep breaths so you can continue to enjoy that good feeling in your ribs.

In the next stretch, you are not only going to continue to give those tight ribs, arms, and shoulders a much-needed stretch, but you will combine it with a stretch of the lower part of your body (see Figure 23).

The two simple stretches in the relaxed position, shown in Figures 22 and 23, can do a great deal to lengthen your body bindings. After several weeks of daily practice, try your full body stretch test again (see Figure 24), and see if your fingers do not come closer to the floor. If they do not, you are not doing your stretches daily and correctly. I guarantee that you will improve if you stay with this simple and effective routine. These stretches, by the way, are most popular with musicians, who need arm and shoulder freedom in their occupation. They can be done anywhere, which is a great advantage when these performers are on the road.

Those who are willing to give a little more attention to the body stretch program but still want to stick to low energy output and nonstrenuous movements can also do the following two exercises (see Figures 25 and 26). Exertion is minimal, and there will be no sweating, but the front of the shoulders and the hip bindings will be much looser.

Shoulders that are hunched forward in chronic poor posture can cause great tightness and stiffness in the chest muscles. So do many athletic activities (volleyball, basketball, golf, and tennis, to name a few) unless they are counteracted by stretches. Free shoulders and hips have a special bonus: the low-back shelf, or sway back, posture can be corrected and a tall, erect look, with high head and centered shoulders, can be reinstated.

For those who are confined to seats for long periods of time, there is a routine that will benefit you without your having to get up. These stretches are good not only for desk workers, but for plane, train, and bus travelers as well. How often have you wanted to take the kinks of out of your torso while flying for several hours? A few good stretches while you are seated can do more for you than running up and down the aisles, especially if you are too tired to even get up and start moving. The intake of more oxygen while stretching is just the lift you will need to build up the energy you need to get going when you arrive at your destination.

For stretches in a plane, train, or bus, you are necessarily limited by the amount of space and the fact that you are seated. But you can still stretch

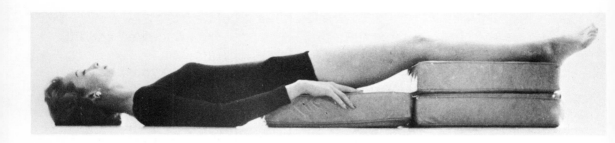

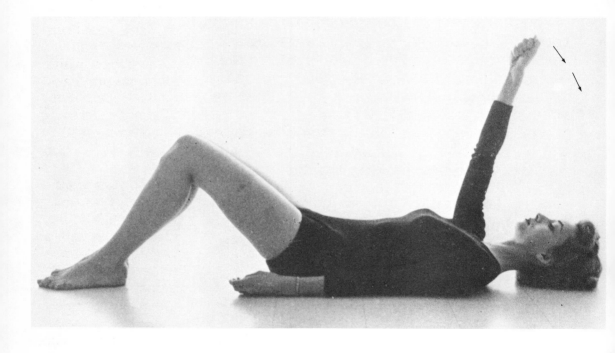

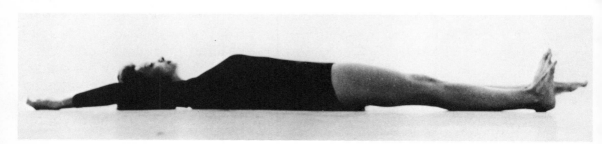

FIGURE 21.
The Full Treatment in Relaxation
For the full treatment in relaxation, *before* stretching, lie on your back (supine). Arrange some cushions so that your hips are higher than your head, and your legs are higher than your hips. Count slowly to 100.

FIGURE 23.
A Full Body Stretch on the Sides
To lift your ribs practically out of your ribcage and at the same time lengthen your leg and pull it strongly at the heel, lie on your back and stretch your right arm back, close to your head. At the same time, stretch your right leg down, *leading with the heel.* Your entire right side should stretch out long. Let go.

Now do the same on the left side, stretching your left arm back close to your head and at the same time stretching your left leg, leading with the heel. Alternate, 10 times on each side.

FIGURE 22.
Arm, Shoulder, and Rib Stretch
Lying on your back with your knees bent, lift your right arm and, keeping it straight, bring it close to your head and stretch it as long and as far back as possible, until you touch the floor. Make your fingers stretch as well. Then let everything loosen and bring your right arm back to your side. Repeat with your left arm. Alternate, stretching each arm 10 times.

In addition to your arms and shoulders, your ribs get a good stretch in this easy movement, provided you surrender all these parts to the movement. It is so seldom the ribs are stretched at all that this one simple stretch feels really good, and both sides need it equally. While you are doing this arm stretch, "speak" to your body and say, "Let go; let go." After 10 stretches for each side, take three deep breaths so you can continue to enjoy that good feeling in your ribs.

FIGURE 24.
Full body Stretch
With your feet together
and your knees straight,
drop forward loosely from
the hips, keeping your
arms relaxed. Bounce
gently three times. Let
your fingertips touch the
floor. Come up slowly.
Repeat. If you can do this
stretch easily, your back
body bindings are entirely
free. As you progress in
the stretching program,
you can test your overall
mobility by assuming this
position (see Figures 2
and 12).

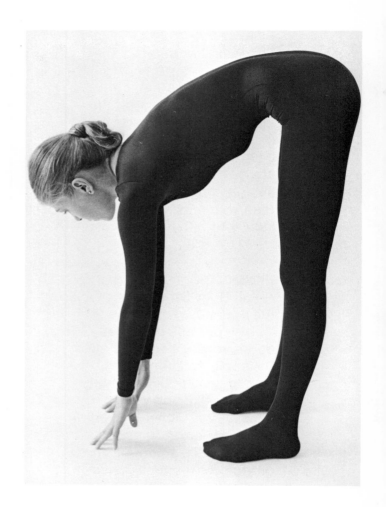

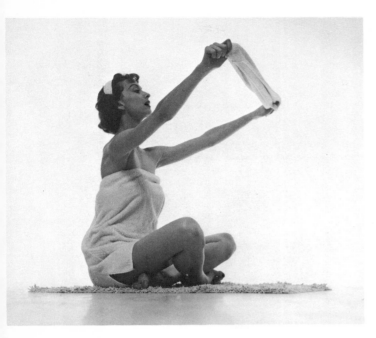

FIGURE 25.
To stretch the bindings in the front of your chest (pectorals), sit on the floor, holding a towel or belt in both hands. Swing the towel overhead, *keeping your elbows straight.* Lower the towel behind your back, making sure to keep your elbows straight all the way.

You will have made a large circle with your arms from front to back, holding the towel all the way. If you feel a pull in the front of the shoulders, you are doing this correctly. Do 10 of these stretches each day.

As your pectoral bindings get looser, bring your hands closer together while holding the towel. After some practice, you will be able to stand tall and place your shoulders where they belong in very good posture. You will feel comfortable and easy, with elasticity and stretchability restored.

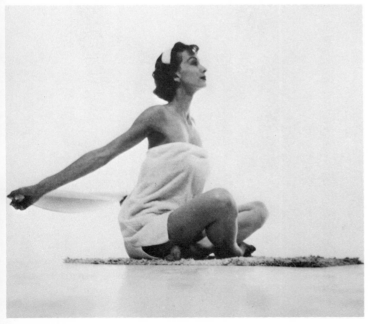

81

FIGURE 26.
An Effective Waist Stretch
for Improved Posture
Place your right hip against
a wall. Keeping it against
the wall, bend sideways,
pulling your right arm over
as far as possible. P–u–l–l.
If you do this correctly,
you will feel the stretch
in your hip.

Come up straight, slowly.
Change sides, placing your
left hip against the wall.
Stretch 3 times on each
side, twice daily.

FIGURE 27.
Sit well back in your seat.
Make sure your hips touch
the back of the seat firmly.
As a matter of fact, your
entire back should touch
the seat back. Keep your
arms directly at your sides.
Without moving your
shoulders or hips from the
back of the seat, drop your
chin as far forward as
possible, imagining that
you are surrendering your
neck. Let it go as loose as
possible.

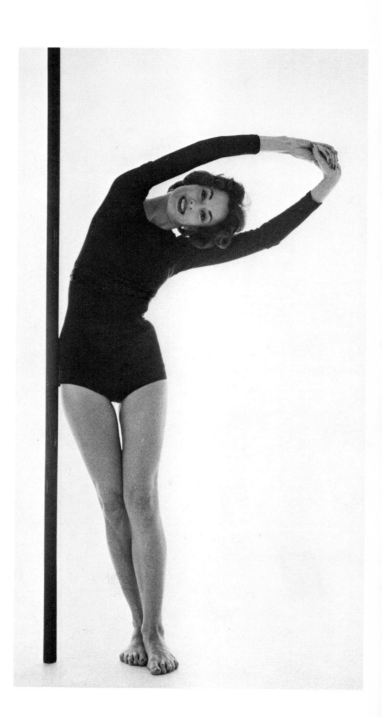

82

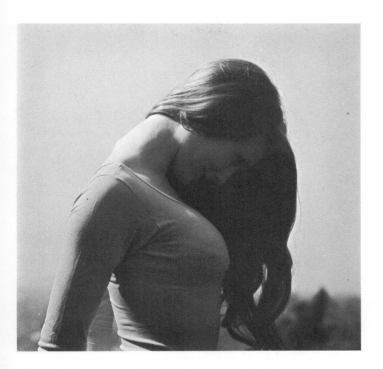

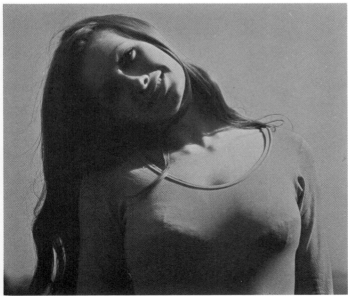

Release your neck easily and bring your head straight up. Repeat this several times.

Look how relaxed the model looks. This simple chin-to-chest movement stretches the bindings where they are tightest for many people.

FIGURE 28.
To loosen the side bindings in your neck, drop your head to the side and bring the tip of your ear to your shoulder. Alternate with each side. Just like the model, surrender your neck so that your head can drop easily and gently to the side as far as possible. If your head cannot go very far, don't be concerned. With practice this will become easier and easier. For those who are particularly tight and stiff in the neck, one of the most effective ways to loosen that part of the body is to stand under a hot shower, with the water flowing directly onto your neck. It is very agreeable to do the neck stretches while under the shower; hot water will prevent any possible soreness in over-tight necks.

FIGURE 29.
Close your eyes and drop your head as far forward as possible; then gently move it to the side as far as possible and roll it way back and over to the other side. You will have made a complete circle with your head.

If you feel little creaks in the back of your neck while you do this, do not be alarmed. These just indicate that your neck needs unkinking, and stretching will help improve circulation while releasing the bindings.

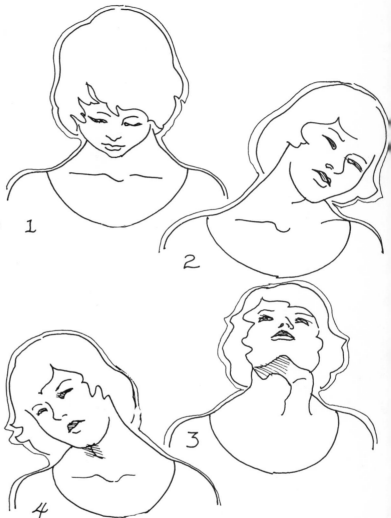

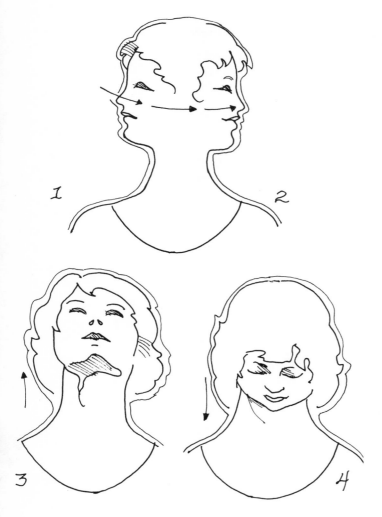

1

2

3

4

FIGURE 30.
It is a good idea to close your eyes and rest them for a bit while traveling. In this position, use the tip of your nose as a pencil and form the letter *T*. Make the cross bar at the top as large as possible; this releases the side neck bindings.

Then draw the letter *O*. Next draw a large letter *E*. Use the tip of your nose and keep your eyes closed. Be sure to keep your shoulders and hips pinned firmly to the seat.

You should regard your head as a large ball on top of a stationary pole—your spine. If your body moves with your head, you lose the useful effect of the stretch.

You should understand this so that your movements are beneficial and effective toward the goal you are working for—the elongation of the neck attachments.

FIGURE 31.

If you are still with this plane, train, or bus routine, there is one more area that needs attention: the front of your neck. Remain seated properly. Drop your head back as far as possible, with your mouth open. With your head still back, close your mouth.

Do you feel a pull at the front of your neck? If you do, you are doing this correctly. Open your mouth again; close it; open it. All the while, your head is back as far as possible. Three of these stretches are sufficient for one sitting.

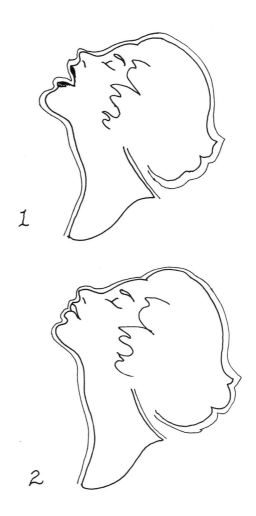

1

2

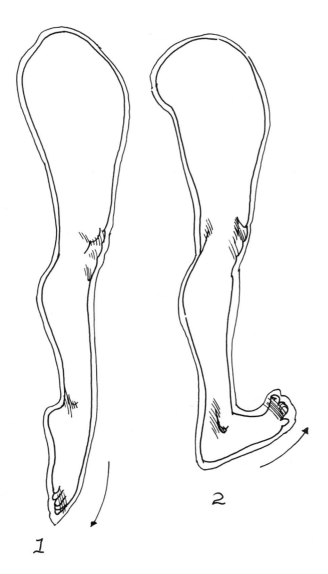

FIGURE 32.
If you are especially ambitious, bored, or full of kinks, you can do leg stretches by straightening your knee and extending your ankle by pointing your toe (a). Then you can extend your heel, all the time keeping your knee straight (b). Relax between each elongation.

1

2

FIGURE 33.
With toe and finger spreads and curls you can give yourself a mild body unkinking with minimal exertion, but it will be a truly beneficial beginning to lenthening bindings.

Stretch out your fingers and toes; then relax them softly. Then simultaneously make a hard fist and curl your toes tightly. Release easily. Repeat 10 times.

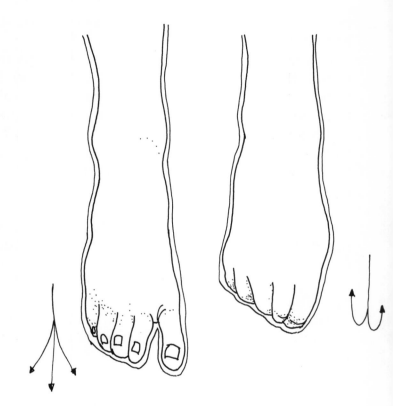

beneficially and help your body bindings loosen (see Figure 27).

Not surprisingly, there are side bindings in addition to the front and back bindings in the neck. Test 1 in Chapter 3 showed you the range of motion in your neck, so you should now appreciate the need to loosen the neck attachments in order to be able to turn your head 90 degrees to each side. You can easily work on this while confined to a desk or airplane (see Figure 28).

As long as you are still sitting in your seat, you can do other effective neck stretches that are relaxing and beneficial for elongating the connections. One is a very soft head roll. Close your eyes and let them go loose while your head rolls around in a circle. This relaxes the eye muscles as well as the neck.

Tension and tightness in the neck are often accompanied by tight jaws. How often have you seen people whose jaws are thrust forward and lips pressed tightly together? This countenance is not only unattractive, but it reflects what the tense person feels.

What a lot of energy is wasted in stiff necks and tight jaws! By loosening these bindings every opportunity you get, you release valuable energy for many other activities.

Try the stretches shown in Figures 29–33. It may not appear that you are doing much in the way of body conditioning, but you have missed the point of this book if you believe in the myth that it takes a sweat-and-toil routine to help the body to better health.

7 Stretches for the Very Active

Very
Active

"Sometimes I exercise just before I go on. I want my whole body to be free."

This is what Benny Goodman, the famous musician said, for like many others, he has discovered the need to have a free body in order to express himself fully.

In the preceding chapters you have learned how to test your own ranges of motion and how to improve the areas that need loosening. Perhaps, to your surprise, you have also discovered that three stretches—a very short but effective routine—can take care of maintenance of body freedom for you. This applies to the healthy person as well as to the clinical patient who has come in with signs of connective tissue erosion and distress. Usually in the latter instance, an individual is willing and anxious to perform whatever routine the medical doctor prescribes; even the most undisciplined, recalcitrant individual will consent to exercises that promise to relieve him of his disturbing symptoms.

Some people may not embrace so eagerly a preventive routine like that advocated and described in Chapter 5. It may be too brief, too repetitive, too routine, to hold the interest of people who are attracted to more complex procedures, more challenging positions, and more intricate movements demanding attention and application. For those who are bored easily, three basic movements may not suffice. It is hoped that the variety introduced here, however, will cause those individuals to extend the time they spend stretching. Those who are in good physical condition, are anxious to maintain that state, and who need a variety of movements to hold their interest can add these new techniques to the basic stretches. It is these individuals to whom this chapter is addressed. The stretches described here will accomplish the same objectives as the three basic movements, but they add variety, complexity, and mobility for the most minute areas of the human structure. The reason for introducing a further variety of stretches has simply to do with the differences in human nature.

These additional stretches are simple enough that they can be done by most people. Those who have had recent illness or injury, however, should obtain medical assurance that they can proceed, although of course this precaution also applies to the basic stretches.

You must remember that the main objective of the stretches is to keep the body free and flexible. Other body conditioning techniques accomplish other goals. Professionals in the field have the knowledge and expertise it takes to achieve the specific goal one desires and needs through body conditioning.

The best way to arrive at a healthy old age minus most bothersome chronic ailments is to take preventive measures in the middle or younger years. Early good health habits prevent illness from taking over later on. Just as there are three tests for range of motion and three stretches to restore that range, there are three R's—right nutrition, restrictions gone, and rest restored—to help prepare you for D-Day: delayed deterioration. If this magic number 3 is too confining, the following stretches can be added to your routine to help you stay loose in all areas.

FIGURE 34.
To stretch the front of your hips and thighs, lie on your stomach (prone) and bend your right leg at the knee. Reach back with both hands and grab your foot, pulling it as far down toward your buttocks as possible. Slowly release. Repeat with your left leg. Stretch three times with each leg.

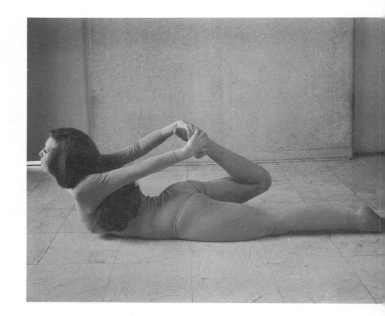

FIGURE 35.
To stretch the back of your hips and thighs, lie on your back and bend your left knee. Reach up and grasp your right leg and, keeping it straight, pull it down toward your chest. Release slowly. Repeat with the opposite leg. Stretch three times with each leg.

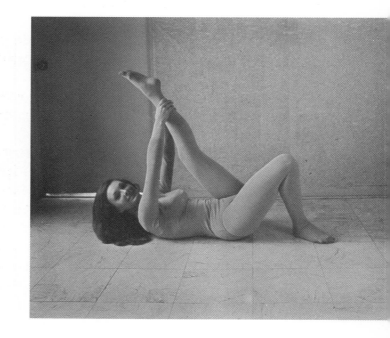

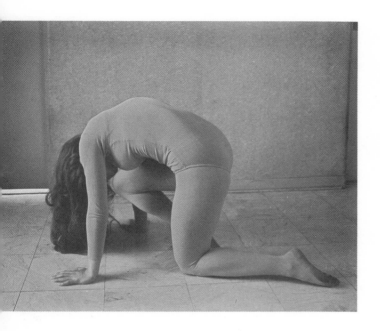

FIGURE 36.
To stretch the front of your hip, get down on all fours and (a) bring your right knee to your forehead. Then (b) shoot the leg straight out and up. Repeat with your left leg. Stretch 10 times with each leg.

(a)

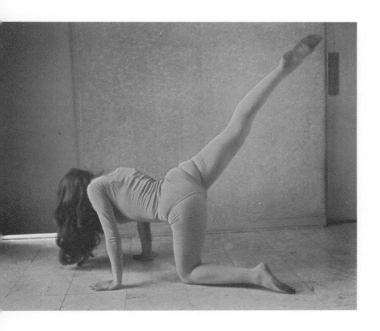

(b)

95

FIGURE 37.
To stretch the lower part of your back, kneel on all fours and (a) raise your spine as high as possible.

Then (b) drop your spine as low as possible. Repeat several times each day.

(a)

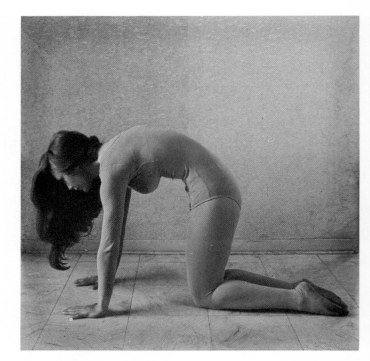

(b)

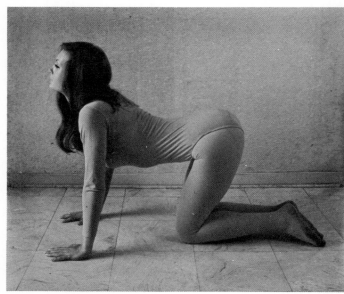

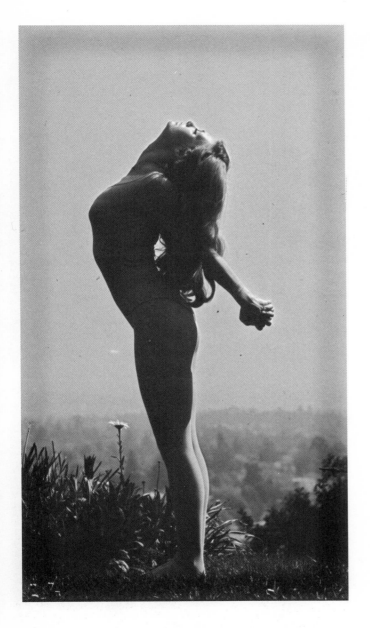

FIGURE 38.
To stretch the bindings in
the front of your neck,
drop your head as far back
as possible and clasp your
hands behind your back.
Keeping your head back,
bring your shoulder blades
as close together as
possible. Release slowly.
Repeat 10 times.

FIGURE 39.
For shoulder flexibility,
reach high in the air, first
with one hand and then
the other, several times a
day.

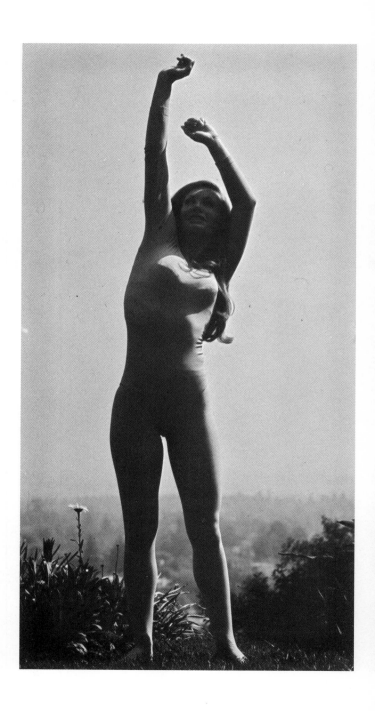

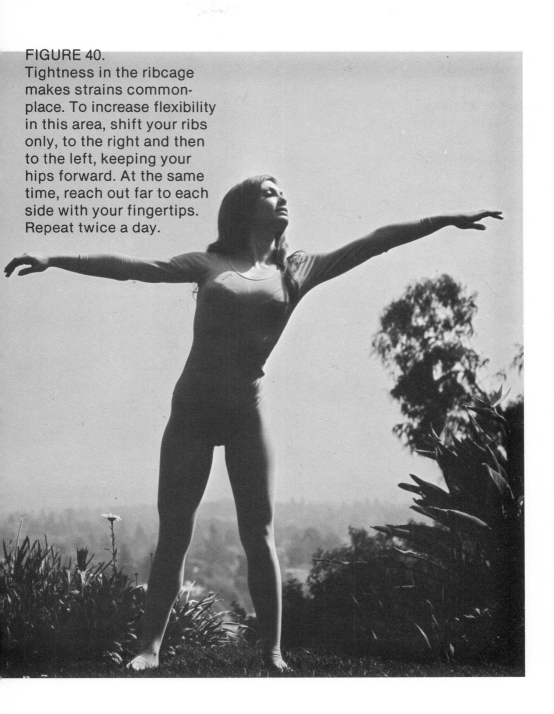

FIGURE 40.
Tightness in the ribcage
makes strains common-
place. To increase flexibility
in this area, shift your ribs
only, to the right and then
to the left, keeping your
hips forward. At the same
time, reach out far to each
side with your fingertips.
Repeat twice a day.

FIGURE 41.
To stretch your waist, clasp your hands and extend your arms far overhead. Stand on one leg and continue to pull your arms upward. You should feel a definite pull. Release and repeat on the opposite side. Stretch 10 times on each side.

Note: Thigh stretches are for the young and those who have stayed youthful.

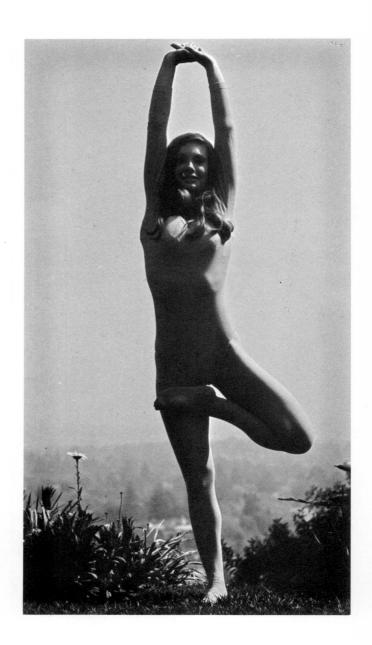

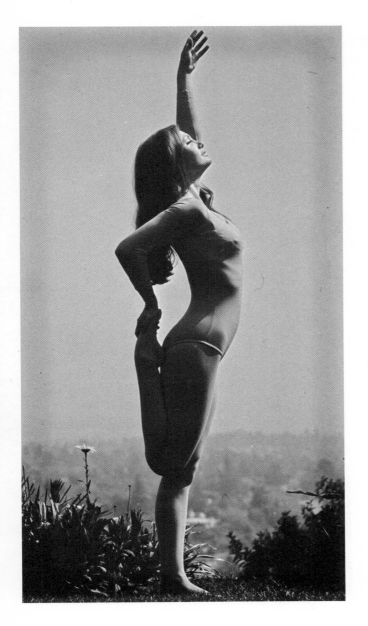

FIGURE 42.
To stretch the front of your thigh, stand on your left leg and reach upward with your left arm. Bend your right leg behind you and hold it with your right hand. Release and repeat on the opposite side. The cross-stretch at the waist and thigh is most effective. Try for five stretches a day and gradually increase.

FIGURE 43.
To stretch the back of your thigh, place your leg on a support in front of you and clasp your arms behind your back. Bend forward slowly, then come up gradually. (This is a more difficult variation of the third basic stretch.) Stretch each leg three times.

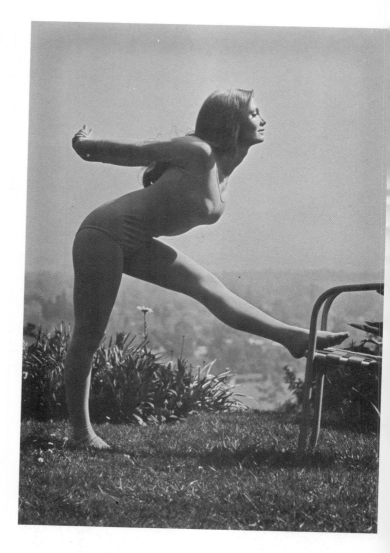

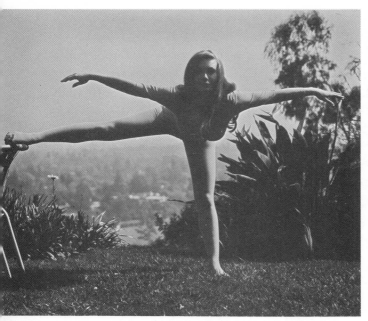

FIGURE 44.
To stretch your inner thigh, place your leg on a support at your side (a) and bend forward slowly, keeping your leg straight out to the side (b). Come up slowly. Stretch each leg three times.

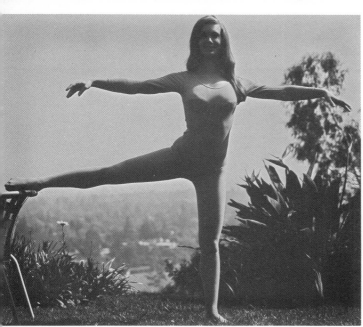

Very
Active

Today, many young athletes are beginning to include agility drills in their body conditioning programs, which heretofore have tended to emphasize other physical attributes. Even powerful athletes like baseball, soccer, and football players are going the stretch route for safety. My most enthusiastic participants in this more active program have been young, active people—dancers, athletes, post-pregnancy cases, and housewives lacking outside physical activity because of household chores.

How much more the rest of us need to pay attention! "Use it or lose it," say the gerontologists. Let us add to that, "No abuse, stay loose."

8 Stretches and Sex

Sex

Are you still young, or thinking young, and your sex life is getting older? Are you liking it less? What can be done for change and/or improvement? In stretching the bindings are we accomplishing anything more than increasing range of motion? Let us examine the evidence.

After many years of treating backaches in a medical clinic, one thing is clear: I have yet to encounter a person in pain or discomfort who is interested in sex at the same time. Pain prevents pleasure seeking, as getting rid of the pain is usually uppermost in the afflicted person's mind. Good health appears to be fundamental to any interest in sex, and pain and stress, both concomitant to a tight body, affect sex.

Of course, certain body restrictions can remain uncorrected and one can engage in sex anyway. But why play "Chopsticks" when you can perform a complete symphony? Some people may not have a choice, but a normal, healthy person does. Normal range of motion is attainable for anybody free of injury or disease.

Let us examine some other facts. The vigor of one's sex function corresponds to the condition of one's general health. Just as the body bindings are free and elastic in youth but gradually lose that elasticity, so other functions of the body, including sex, will normally slacken as a person gets older or neglects them. The person who expects to perform at the level of a 20-year old for a lifetime is as unrealistic as a champion prizefighter who expects to maintain his title until he is 50 years of age or more. There are rare exceptions, however. Body functions in general taper off in strength and vitality, but they do so very slowly and imperceptibly in some and more markedly in others. When there is a sudden decline or premature absence of sex, however, one should consult the experts, as there may be help. It is a complicated subject and one that has been tackled by many disciplines.

It is important to understand some of the more common facts about sex. Sex has a strange quality quite different from other body functions. Other organs, such as the stomach, liver, and lungs, cannot cease to function for any length of time without damaging the body in some way, and when one of these organs does malfunction, life-saving methods must be applied to keep the person alive. Not so with sex. This function can be put to rest and it can remain at rest without destroying other vital functions of the body. Life goes on even without sex. Some persons choose this way of life, but others do not.

Another fact about life and sex has come to the fore more recently. With freer discussions and personal revelations on the subject, it has become apparent that sex interest and sexual expression extend throughout life. In other words, sex is not only for the young; the elderly want it too. With our cultural emphasis on youth in sex and romance, the revelation that sex continues throughout life is more of a shock for the young than the old.

An 80-year old patient in a senior facility announced one day that she was going to go modern that night. "I'm going to streak," she announced when asked what she planned to do. Her dash through the main lobby in her birthday suit that evening made history in the home, not to mention the conversations that ensued. The intense gossip of her fellow inhabitants released many a suppressed desire.

What connection is there between stretches and sex? When you consider that sex positions depend upon the agility of your body, on the freedom of all body bindings to release and yield the various segments, you can deduce very quickly that a tight body in various sex positions is only going to cause a lot of clumsiness and pain, not to mention cramps, a very common complaint of adults in clinics over the years. From a functional point of view, this is not surprising. The inner thighs and inner pelvic muscle attachments are not used very much in daily life. Their use can be traced back to a much earlier period in man's history when he climbed trees for food to sustain life. Then the inner muscles and their attachments had to be free and easy so that they could function efficiently. If we are not athletes or performers but just ordinary humans who walk daily, the inner thighs and pelvis will tighten up considerably over the years. This is a common condition. To spread the legs, to assume the exotic postures so explicitly illustrated in Asian, Indian, and now Western art, it will take elongation of the inner thigh and pelvic bindings for those over 35.

To relieve the cramps and become more mobile, the side fling illustrated in Figure 45 is recommended. If you surrender your leg and try to achieve a complete 90-degree angle in your stretching, you will be on your way to crampless interludes.

The act of sex not only calls for mobility of the body but for muscle strength and endurance as well, and these are directly dependent upon the yieldability of the body bindings. When the bindings are

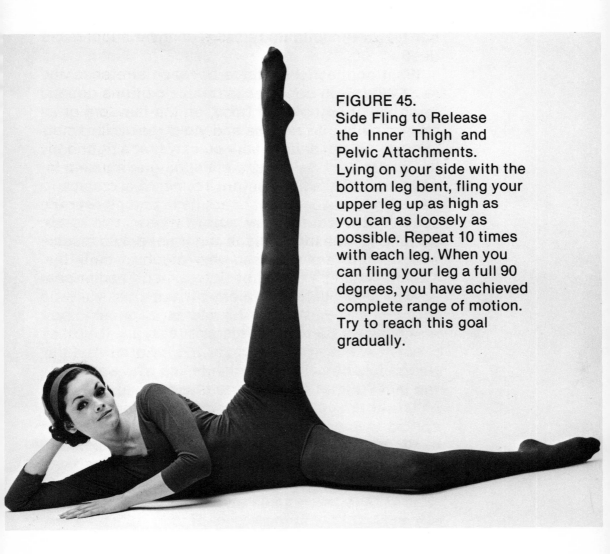

FIGURE 45.
Side Fling to Release
the Inner Thigh and
Pelvic Attachments.
Lying on your side with the
bottom leg bent, fling your
upper leg up as high as
you can as loosely as
possible. Repeat 10 times
with each leg. When you
can fling your leg a full 90
degrees, you have achieved
complete range of motion.
Try to reach this goal
gradually.

elastic and elongated, they permit the muscle bundles encased in fibrous tissue to expand and contract to their fullest capacity and, consequently, to their best advantage. Optimal strength and endurance would be possible with optimal binding flexibility. A tight encasement, on the other hand, would restrict muscle action, and muscle function and efficiency would be reduced. Premature muscle fatigue would affect strength and endurance in the sex act.

When doctors advise couples whose sex life is lagging to take vacations in order to restore sexual interest and compatibility, physical and mental relaxation is the restorative ingredient. This means yield of body bindings, yield of thoughts, yield of desire—in other words, total release. Stretching can also break the tension cycle and relieve feelings of stress. There are other avenues to relaxation, but the physical approach is so simple, so available, and one that you can readily understand and appreciate. With a little application, your body will say "Thank you" very quickly.

Sometimes a person's problem is not tension but tight body bindings caused by other factors (see Chapter 4). Let us examine two cases and the effects of body bindings on sex. Sam was 50 years of age and had sought medical help for a backache. He was a married man with several children but no longer had intercourse with his wife. He had just returned from a business trip to Rio with a 28-year-old girlfriend, who accompanied him. His tight back had bothered him before he left, but upon his return the pain had increased markedly, and he needed instant relief. A complete medical examination showed no pathology (bone or joint deterioration), but a physical evaluation showed marked restriction of all his body bindings, particularly in the hip area. Any bending forward from the waist down was sharply cut off. His fingertips stopped above his knees (Figure 2).

His young partner was able to delight him sexually since she had all the elasticity and agility it took to pleasure him. Any attempts on his part to become the vigorous, active, and thrusting male he was formerly were met with kinks, stiffness, and knifelike reminders from his hips, which were registering an angry protest. He volunteered this information in his medical history because he was more concerned about being a satisfactory sex partner in the future than he was in getting rid of his back problem. He learned, however, that the two problems were actually one. If he had free-swinging hips, the painful kinks would be gone. The rest he could take care of himself and did.

Another patient, Joe, a bachelor, was 55 and had the rigidity of a wooden Indian. Back pains were beginning to bother him, and he was referred for treatment of low-back pain and for a complete physical evaluation. All of his body bindings were like steel cables. You could feel the hard cords at the back of his neck and the sides of the knees, where the bindings attach to the bone.

When questioned about his physical activities, he replied that outside of sex he had none. And even sex called for only minimal motion as he described the following. Being a bachelor and coming from a highly repressed background, he had been timid early in life about forming relationships with females. He had never married and had known only paid sex partners throughout his adult life. He would lie passively and allow his hired provider to service him sexually. He had started this way in his early youth and never changed in 30 years. With only minimal joint motion, stretching, turning, and minimal use of his own muscle strength for thrusting, he had arrived at the point of overshortened body bindings. All ranges of motion were excessively limited. A complete mobilization program was necessary to restore any flexibility. Any stretch activities had to counteract the passive, supine positions he had maintained over many years because he had had practically no physical activities of any kind to counteract body rigidity. He had developed rigor mortis-like joints long before his time. He had not used stretches to delay his body's deterioration.

These two cases, so explicit as to the connection between body mobility and sex, are typical of hundreds of similar cases illustrating the relationship between body mobility, range of motion, muscle capacity, and sex.

Hip tightness can be tested separately, even more specifically than in Test 3 in Chapter 3, where you learned to pinpoint tightness from the waist down (see Figure 46).

A simple, undemanding stretch done daily will lengthen the bindings in the lower back. Most orthopedists recommend it to alleviate low back pain. It is a gentle stretch but in spite of its seeming simplicity, it does the job. (Again, check with your medical doctor first if you have any history of injury, disease, or back trouble for which you needed medical care. Stretches are for those who are completely healthy.)

Simply pressing your lower back down to the floor while supine is a gentle starter for hip stretching (see Figure 47). In addition, performing the knee press (see Figure 48), also while lying on your back, stretches the center part of your hips, and the knee drop (Figure 49) stretches the sides of your hips. Such a stretching routine, done twice a day, 10 times each stretch, can restore swing and sway in your hips and assure complete comfort and enjoyment in any activities requiring hip movement thereafter, including sex.

To check your own improvement, return to the wall and repeat the test shown in Figure 46 to see if you can now accomplish what was difficult before. Can you pin your lower back to the wall? Is your entire back flat against the wall? If you can do this easily and comfortably, you have the normal range of motion desirable for sex without limits or painful cramps.

Since body bindings and muscles are so intimately tied to the physical aspects of sex, my dealings with polio patients in a medical clinic provided an excellent opportunity to learn more about the role these structures played in sex and the changes that had to take place after the destruction of the muscles. In rehabilitating the polio victim, we turned our attention to the restoration not only of his physical function but his total personality. What could be done to give him the aid and support he needed to allow the full expression of his own unique being? This led us to an in-depth study of the sex life of the polio victim. The case histories and revelations of that study were to be added to the volume Dr. Alfred C. Kinsey was preparing. It was a special study of

FIGURE 46.
Place your back to a wall
with your head, shoulders,
and hips touching. Keep
your heels about two
inches away from the wall.
You are now standing
perfectly straight; however,
the lower part of your
spine will be slightly
curved away from the wall.
This is normal.

Without moving any part
away from the wall, flatten
the lower part of your spine
against the wall. Can you
touch the wall with your
entire spine, including the
lower part, without moving
your shoulders or hips
away from the wall?

If you can, then there is
enough yield in your body
bindings to allow freedom
of movement in your hips.
If not, and there is a hollow
present, your hip bindings
are tight and need to be
loosened. Fortunately, it is
not difficult to correct.

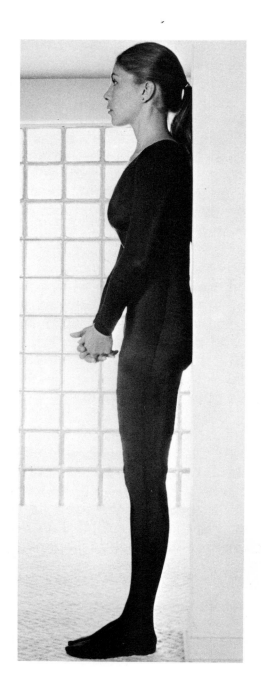

114

FIGURE 47.
To have a slight curve in
your lower back is normal,
provided that you can
stretch it flat to the floor
without moving any other
part of the body. To
lengthen the lower back
bindings in order to be
able to do this comfortably,
press your lower back to
the floor 10 times, twice a
day.

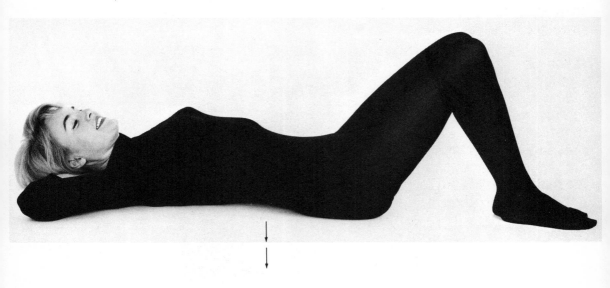

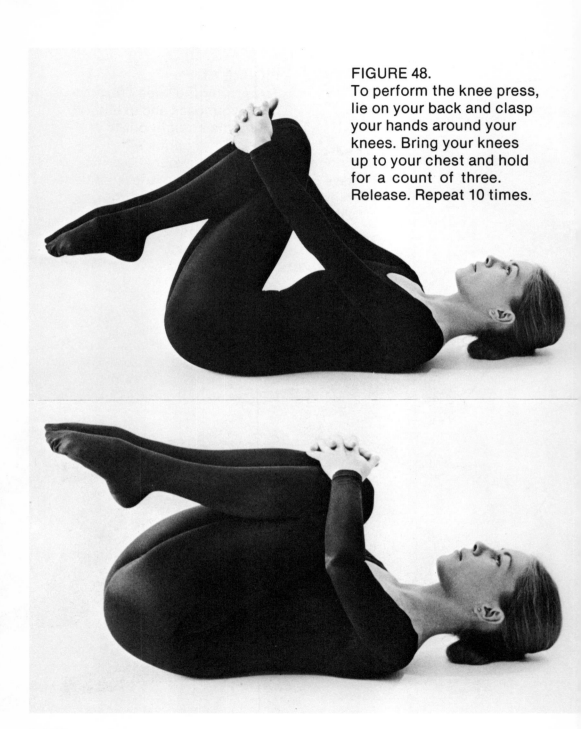

FIGURE 48.
To perform the knee press,
lie on your back and clasp
your hands around your
knees. Bring your knees
up to your chest and hold
for a count of three.
Release. Repeat 10 times.

FIGURE 49.
To perform the knee drop,
lie on your back and extend
your arms straight out to
the sides at shoulder
height. Bring your knees
up, keeping them together,
and drop them to the right.
Bring them back up and
drop them to the left.
Repeat 10 times.

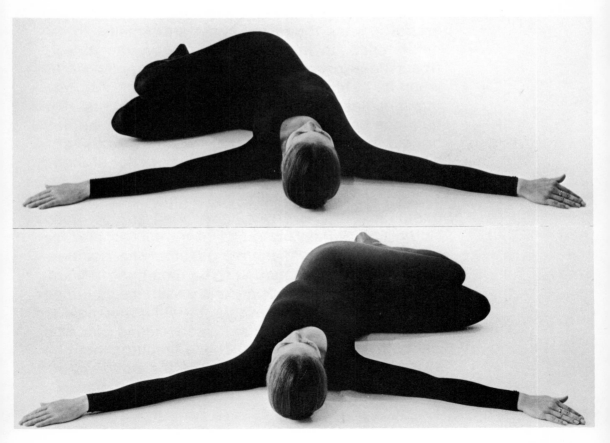

the sex life of the handicapped, and it remained un-published because of his sudden death.

A few myths concerning sex and related activities emerged from this study and are of interest in the context of stretch reflexes. Polio is not contagious after the incubation period, so sex is not "out" but can continue with certain modifications of technique. Healthy children can be born by a polio-stricken mother.

The fact that the affected muscle loses its power to move, however, condemns that particular body part to immobility. Remember the example of the student who had his arm bound in a sling and at the end of a week found his lower arm smaller in circumference. In much the same way, the muscle fibers deteriorate and atrophy in the polio victim when he or she can no longer move them. Atrophying muscles then begin to affect the joints. The bindings begin to assume the position they are left or held in. You will recall that the elbow of the student whose arm was in the sling would not straighten out completely after the sling was removed because the bindings had become stiff. Thus, we can understand the overwhelming need of the polio victim to maintain his range of motion so that his body does not permanently assume one position, which usually is seated with the hips bent forward. If his pelvis, because of muscle weakness, is tipped forward like a bowl, he eventually will not be able to straighten it again because the shortened bindings will hold it tipped forward. These bindings must be stretched out and in the case of the polio victim, the elongation is performed by a medical therapist.

One of the best and easiest methods to keep your joints mobile for complete range of motion is swimming. The daily pool activities that President Franklin Delano Roosevelt engaged in over many years contributed to his ability to maintain range of motion in all areas of his body and consequently enabled him to use whatever musculature remained. According to recent reports about his intimate life, he remained sexually active until quite late in life.

Pool therapy is not only for post-polio patients, however. It is a convenient medium for stretching. If you are one of those who finds it difficult to learn to let go, the pool is a good place to work on loosening your joints. Water also removes gravity, and its buoyancy allows you to float with ease. Water lovers can benefit from body improvement when land maneuvering is too difficult or uncomfortable, as in the case of the handicapped. Simple, gentle, nonhazardous stretches in the pool have particular appeal not only to the handicapped, who cannot stretch on land without aid, but to other, nonhandicapped people who are inactive or elderly. A 72-year-old grandmother would not miss her daily swim. She was taught the breast stroke, which stretches the front of the shoulders, to benefit her shoulders and arms, which were cupped forward from 40 years of bending over a piano to teach children how to play. She also does the back stroke, which helps stretch her tight rib-cage and front shoulders. Her shortened bindings have been helped greatly by the daily swims.

For others, the stretching of their legs and the front of their hips that comes with swimming is a welcome change from the sedentary posture that caused the overshortening in the first place. Another stretch that can be done in the pool is hanging by your hands from a diving board for a count of 10. This provides a full body stretch. It cannot be repeated often enough that if you maintain one body position for too long without any efforts to counteract it, it is going to take its toll with excessive shortening of the bindings. This can be avoided, of course, and if sex is your interest, it is advisable to remain entirely mobile in order to enjoy the pleasure of a highly colorful and varied repertoire.

In our study of the changes of sex techniques of married polio victims, we learned of the tremendous importance of the hip muscles and their bindings in both males and females. When these were affected, the unaffected partner would have to take all the action so that the affected partner could achieve orgasm. When the hip muscles were not involved, however, the sex techniques could remain almost the same. A patient who had one arm completely paralyzed and the other partially paralyzed could no longer embrace her husband during sex. This called for adjustment that she stated was not too difficult: mobilization of the shoulder joints still continued. Another patient, however, a male whose hip muscles and bindings still had normal range but whose legs and one arm had residual paralysis, had to assume a side-lying position to be effective. This was a new posture for him.

A female patient's front hip and lower extremities were paralyzed, and this ruled out her favorite sex position. She preferred to lie prone while her husband mounted her from the rear, but because of her polio and the resultant shortening of her hip bind-ings, she could no longer assume that posture with comfort or ease; it was too painful. Needless to say, we tried to aid her with mobilization to elongate the tissues.

Clearly it is important to avoid the excessive shortening of body bindings so you can participate in all activities with comfort and ease, including sex. Maintaining ranges of motion or restoring former flexibility is the answer.

9 For The Sports Minded

Sports
Minded

Dr. Black, a very busy dentist extremely devoted to his practice, could not turn his head from side to side without considerable pain, which radiated down his arm all the way to his wrist. His weekly golf games seemed to aggravate his pain. How come? He always thought that activity was good for him, so why didn't it help his neck and arm? He was frightened. Would he have to give up dentistry? It was becoming more painful for him to practice each day. Would he have to drop golf? What kind of life was this? With such worries, his tension and pain rose to an excruciating level, and that brought him to the medical clinic. By the time he arrived, he was suffering from an intolerable spasm. Laboratory tests and medical examinations revealed no disease processes. What was the explanation for all his suffering?

In spite of the newest equipment, dentists must work in a constantly stooped-forward position. Their necks, shoulders, and arms are continuously contracted, and they have very little time between patients to rest and relax the body bindings and muscles. When the bindings are held in constant contraction day in and day out with only a two-week vacation once a year (if that); tensions build up, and the bindings are going to complain. In addition, Dr. Black was an avid golfer and played weekly. This sport calls for emphasis on the same body parts as in dentistry. The one great difference, however, is that the golfer must release the body bindings to make a good swing. How can he release them properly when they are already overtight and remain shortened even while he's swinging? Swinging with tight bindings will ultimately cause stress signals. This is the dilemma.

Recently, I observed a golfer driving his ball hard but achieving just average distance. Naturally he was disturbed.

"My drives are so bad," he complained. "It's all because I had a heart attack that my game has gone to pot."

"How long is it since you have given your body a good stretching?" I asked.

"Oh, I haven't done exercises for years. The doctor did not say anything about stretching. He just said I should golf nine holes once a week for exercise."

Even an untrained eye could observe what was wrong with this man's swing. It was stiff, inelastic, shortened, and tense. No wonder he could not make mileage with the ball. Years of tightening and tension had shortened his body bindings, restricting his range of motion for swinging. His joint restrictions came out in his golf game, and his joints would become even stiffer if neglected over time. His heart condition would no doubt improve with walking, but his anger and subsequent tension at his deteriorating golf game would counteract any improvement. Anger-engendered tension is a first-class enemy to body health. It may quicken muscle energy and mental alertness, but the strain on vital processes more than offsets any other advantages.

The dentist's case called for a complete body mobilization program in order for him to continue practicing dentistry and playing golf. He would be able to do both with ease and comfort, but only after a head-to-toe loosening for 10 minutes each morning and the same later in the day. A daily routine was imperative for the program to be effective.

During the first week of body stretching nothing changed. The dentist was disappointed, but he was reminded that it took 20 years for his body to get where it was today, with stiffness and tightness, and it was going to take more than one week of stretching to restore his original body flexibility. After approximately four weeks, his bindings began to give noticeably. We checked his progress by having him bend forward and try to touch the floor (see Figure 2). Initially, before treatment, the dentist's fingertips stopped 25 inches off the floor. In his improved condition, he could extend them down to 6 inches off the floor. A gain of 19 inches worth of body flexibility had been achieved. Although that was a good result, even better could be attained with additional application.

Some persons stretch out quickly, and others take longer. Full body mobility is only the beginning for the athlete who wants to improve his game, but the body must be completely mobile before he can concentrate on refining his play.

A very active woman in her sixties, who was scheduled to play in a professional tennis match the following day, became alarmed. Her playing elbow was aching severely (tennis elbow), and she wanted an instant cure. She certainly didn't want to hear that her practice would have to be moderate or even sparing until the elbow distress subsided. What made the situation even more threatening was the woman's occupation. She was a sculptor and was in the middle of preparing an exhibit. Like the dentist, the overuse of a body part in her occupation and in her chosen sport was inviting trouble. The overuse of a body part can cause it to deteriorate just as much as its underuse. Mobility of neck and shoulder muscles had to be restored with only moderate tennis playing until her sculpting exhibit was completed.

The first point of attention for the sportsminded, then, is to note what your occupation does to your body. Does your job force you to keep your head leaning forward and your shoulders cupped? Are you seated all day at a desk, typewriter, cash register, etc.? The process of overshortening may not be noticeable in those between 20 and 30 years old, but after 35 it becomes evident. The accumulated tightness can become severely aggravated by 40, and the longer the tightness is neglected, the longer and harder effort it will take to counteract it. So staying loose is the first step toward any athletic improvement.

Each sport involves a specific part of the body, and that is the part that should function particularly well for an athlete to improve his scores and competence. But handball, tennis, and golf all call for use of the same set of joints and bindings that are shortened when one remains sedentary. The tightness and tension engendered in one's occupation may be aggravated by the person's activity program unless the bindings involved are elongated.

Before going into more detail on how to achieve even better performance, however, we should take a look at several athletes and performers who are presently attracting attention by doing extraordinary things. If they were not completely mobile at all junctures of their bodies, they could not even attempt to perform the stunts that they do. This group of people includes dancers, football players, figure skaters, and free-style skiers, just to name a few, and their activities require complete mobility of all bindings, including those in the inner thighs and pelvis (see Chapter 8).

The deterioration and the overshortening of the body bindings as a result of inactivity was so prominent in the clinic scene that we felt compelled to check this out with the sportsminded. How basic is body flexibility to athletic performance? How important for the average player? For the champion?

In the field of tennis, there are no authorities superior to the Sutton family. May Sutton, the mother of Dorothy Cheney, who is now carrying the tournament torch for the Sutton clan, was the first overseas winner of the Wimbledon championship in 1905, and she repeated her success in 1907. Her phenomenal record has rightfully earned her the title of "Woman Athlete of the Century." Her first tournament win was at the age of 12 and her last was at the age of 85 (see Figure 50)! This is not an easy record to beat. Her daughter Dorothy, better known as Dodo, has been ranked among the top 10 U.S. women champions for 10 years, and she is continuing to chalk up championships to equal her illustrious mother.

May Sutton's Wimbledon wins took place during the era of corsetted waists and frilly petticoats, even on the tennis court. That restrained, genteel type of game disappeared completely with the Suzanne Lenglen–Helen Wills matches in 1926 and later. Women's tennis evolved into the high-powered game with blazing serves and powerful slugs that we know today.

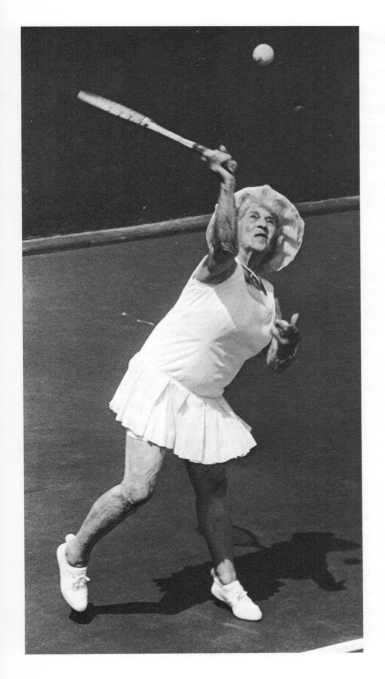

FIGURE 50.
May Sutton, the only woman tennis champion and athlete in this century who actively followed her favorite sport for over 70 years after achieving top world honors.

Courtesy *Evening Outlook:* photo by Bob Smith

Sports Minded

"When you lay off for six weeks, you become less elastic," replied Dorothy Cheney when questioned about possible stiffness from inactivity. "You must stretch out again, but you also must do it gradually. Take it easy at first, don't play too hard—just take it easy playing two or three times a week so that you can maneuver completely again. This is very important. Otherwise, you can pull a muscle.

"When I have strained an elbow or knee, I play it out on the court. I go very easy. Some persons are put into a sling, however, and others have to quit altogether until the pain goes away." When asked what brought these strains on, she agreed that tension at the joints caused the difficulty in most cases. When I asked if staying loose was a good guideline for tennis playing, Dorothy agreed heartily. "By all means, that is the key to good tennis—stay maneuverable."

"How else can you help a person improve his game?" I asked.

She offered four suggestions that would be helpful to any tennis player, amateur or professional:

1) Practice, practice, and more practice. This seems to be true in doing well at anything. Repetition and total involvement make skills stick.

2) Play with a player better than yourself as often as possible. This way you must become totally involved and you improve your concentration.

3) Participate in as many tournaments as possible. Dorothy believes that competition provides a good training ground for emotional stability. A person playing in a tournament is confronted with many emotions so that when the big matches come around, emotional maturity can stand one in good stead.

4) The most important point is to stay in good physical shape. Maintain complete flexibility, making sure that all joints are free and have complete range of motion.

"Short warm-ups before games can be too brief," she said, "particularly on a cold morning outdoors. Tight hips and knees will cut down springing action in footwork, and tense shoulders and elbows will throw off timing in serves and strokes. When your timing is off, you are hitting the ball too late or too soon. You must be totally relaxed and released to hit the ball at the peak of the bounce and have perfect timing."

Why do champion players make it look so easy? What does it take to achieve their success? We have all had the experience of participating in a six-course holiday dinner for 10 prepared by a host or hostess with such grace, speed, and ease that it seems to the uninitiated like there is nothing to it, that anyone can do it. Watching championship matches may also give the false impression that such skill is easy to accomplish. Experts in any endeavor always make it look so easy. That is why they are experts.

The organization, practice, and skill that go into planning, preparing, and serving the dinner are much the same as the effort required to achieve superior performance in a game of skill like tennis. Tension, poor timing, lack of expertise, and lack of body maneuverability all contribute to the poor performance of a beginner. The skillful performance, on the other hand, comes with complete lack of both physical and mental tension, omission of excess motion, excellent timing, months and months of back-up practice, and that extra ingredient: joy of performance.

"Why do I run almost every day of the year, in rain, snow, and heat waves? Only because I love running," explained Joan Ullyot, women's marathon world record holder.

Now that you have the secret recipe from the mouths of the champs, you can set about improving your score. One thing that should impress you deeply is that staying loose is the single most important part of physical fitness.

Those who wish to improve their golf scores should apply the same principles that are important in tennis. The power of concentration is mentioned frequently; this cuts out extraneous motion and improves the strokes.

For the beginner, the position of the golf club as an extension of the arm feels awkward, but it becomes more comfortable with practice. He or she simply has to become accustomed to it. In addition, although head turning ordinarily goes with arm lifting, and this is a reflex built-in since infancy, in golf, the head must be held down while the arms and shoulders move. This too has to be learned, although it is often difficult. Even long-time golfers must remind themselves to keep their heads down. A conscious effort must be made, but with frequent practice, it can be learned. Concentration, practice, repetition, and relaxing the part of the body not involved in swinging goes into training the body for good golf swings. Tension, awkwardness, and poor timing all prevent good scoring, particularly for the beginner.

Notice that again tension heads the list. Unabated, it can lead to a vicious cycle for the player, who then may have great difficulty ever achieving better scores. When the body is tight, the bindings are the parts of the structure that contract. With contraction the bindings and their attachments become shortened and cut down the arc of swinging. Abruptly interrupted with an unpleasant tug, the swing tends to become shorter and shorter, and a vicious cycle of shortening and irritation is set off. Tension also restricts your movement; and timing, efficiency of movement, and power of application all are affected by restriction. A program of stretches for body freedom, however, will improve the score, so stay loose.

Let us check out another source of professional expertise. Duckie Drake, 30 years a master trainer of world-famous Olympic athletes, coach of Rafer Johnson and C. K. Yang, first- and second-place decathalon winners in Rome, knows some fundamental points for the sportsminded.

"What do you consider the best exercises for golf or tennis players, particularly for those who are no longer youngsters?" I queried.

"Stretches, stretches, and more stretches," he replied. "It is one of the best conditioning exercises no matter what sport or activity. Of course, I do recommend walking, then pacing, then light jogging. This must be gradual—also the stretches. A little at a time, then gradually building up."

Since Duckie is an excellent golfer, I asked what suggestions he had for improving golf scores.

"Keep your head down," he answered quickly. This seems to be one of the most difficult things to learn, especially for the beginner.

133

Drake offered another suggestion. "Don't forget stretches in golf. You want to finish at the top of your swing. To get a good long, easy, wide swing, you have to be loose in the arms and shoulders. That's where your stretches count. Swing high and finish at the top, not at the back of the head as so many do. That cuts your ball to the side."

Since Duckie comes into contact with many strains and pulled muscles, he is well aware of the need for complete range of body motion at all times, and in all ages, including young trainees now under his tutelage for new championships.

"To be stretched out keeps injuries down," he observed. I asked him how we could make our bodies last longer for full enjoyment of sports. "Well, keep fit, keep healthy and, above all, think young."

Thirty years head trainer at UCLA, a school known for its renowned athletes, Drakes keeps pushing his own skills. He personally illustrates the fact that the older a person gets, the more he has to reinforce sports skills to keep them alive. A 25-year-old can take a break from tennis or golf for a couple of months and resume playing at his former level of skill after a few rusty sessions, but a 62-year-old cannot. He must continue to practice in order to remain active and maintain his expertise.

Observing Duckie Drake, you see a living example of a man who has maintained physical skills far beyond the middle years. He keeps pushing, remains active, and thinks young. That formula will improve anybody's score.

Duckie and I heartily agree that free lower extremities are essential in sports activities. He has a favorite stretch for the heel cord (see Figure 51). It is one

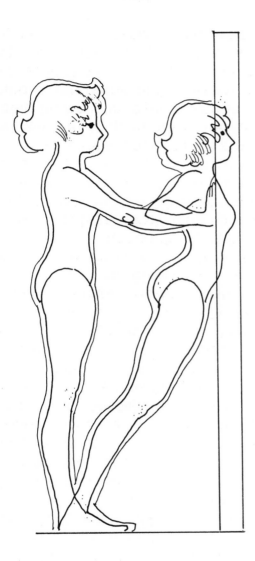

FIGURE 51.
Heel Cord Stretch
Stand at arm's distance facing a wall or open doorway. Extend your arms in front of you and lean forward, placing your hands on the wall or on either side of the doorway. Keeping your heels well back, slowly lower your chest to the wall or through the doorway, depending on where you are doing the stretch.

Be sure not to bend, but keep your back and knees straight. If you feel a pull at your heels, you are doing the stretch correctly. The farther your heels are from the wall, the more your lower extremities are being stretched.

As you improve, gradually increase the distance of your heels from the wall.

that was taught in school many years ago, and it works if done correctly.

For even better results, try Stretch 3 in Chapter 5. Do this fundamental low back and heel cord stretch, and if you feel a decided tug at your hips, knees, or heels, you need to elongate your lower extremities.

Here are some additional suggestions to assist the sportsminded:

- A short daily workout is more beneficial than longer workouts on weekends only.
- Warm up before any workouts. Swing your racket or club lazily at first, and then build up to full range and stronger effort.
- Wear a protective covering to keep from getting chilled while perspiring. Notice that the champions immediately put on sweaters or warm jackets after competition.
- While you are perspiring, do not go into air-conditioned areas. Sudden chilling and body tightening are a "gruesome twosome."
- A prolonged hot bath takes out any soreness from too-severe workouts.
- Overweight tummies drag on the lower back bindings. Try to get rid of the bulge to relieve the constant pull.
- Keep going to keep your skills alive, especially in later years.

Although you may be aware of all of these hints and suggestions, it may be a good idea to review them once in a while to refresh your memory.

10 Heads Up— You Win

Heads UP

Posture is very much like the weather. It is always there. It is the sum total of all your movements throughout your entire life, and it includes static positions as well as activity. It is your body at rest and your body in motion. The way you move or stand has a direct bearing on your body's physiological functioning. If function is poor, it can be related to poor posture. Unfortunately, most of us learn this in the middle years, when there is still time to correct the faults but it is more difficult than if we had been aware of them earlier in life. Habits of 30 years or more can be changed, but the challenge is very great. The fewer the years of habit, the easier a problem is to correct.

It is most fitting to discuss posture when speaking of the body's range of motion—the main theme of this book. Good posture is entirely dependent upon range of motion. Without it you cannot carry your head high—right on top of your spine, where it belongs (see Figure 52). You cannot lengthen your spine to an elongated mild "S" curve. You cannot place your pelvis directly under the base of your spine. Your knees will not be directly under your hips, and your feet will not move in an easy parallel position. In other words, your body parts will be out of line (see Figure 53).

Your assignment, then, is to get your body segments into line. Your ligaments will then be relieved of the pounding they receive when your body segments are out of line.

What are some of the more common things that cause the body to get out of line?

When children are young, great care should be exercised by parents and teachers in choosing posture cues. Telling children to stand up like soliders or policemen, to put their shoulders back, or suck in their tummies all lead to stiff, exaggerated positions. Children could unconsciously carry this over into adult life. Other cues are more helpful. Telling them to stand tall with their heads up, to relax their shoulders, and to keep their feet parallel when walking are only a few.

Let's start at the top and look at the position of your head. One of the most common faults in aging posture is to drop the head and the neck forward. This causes a protuberance of the lower neck bones called a "widow's hump." In early times the many years a widow spent with her head bowed in mourning brought on this name. But this posture problem is not found only in older people. Through bad habits or sedentary occupations young people practice the same faulty body mechanics. It is avoidable, however.

"My isn't she stunning?"

"Yes, she looks better in person than any photograph. She is positively beautiful."

You may not believe that this was said of a very tall, plain-featured, older woman of great fame, Eleanor Roosevelt; yet it was. Why?

At no time, even well into her later years, did she abandon the youthful carriage of her head and neck. They were always held erect, sitting majestically on a long graceful spine, which was also erect. When interviewed, she confessed to early good posture training, and obviously she never lost it.

To carry your head high on top of your spine, to stretch your neck long and tall, and to square your shoulders straight out at the side takes years off

FIGURE 52.
Standing Posture
Good body alignment
means that all body parts
are in an optimum position
in relation to gravity. If a
gravity line were drawn,
it would pass through the
lobe of the ear, the tip of
the shoulder, the center of
the hip joint, the back of
the knee cap, and just in
front of the ankle.

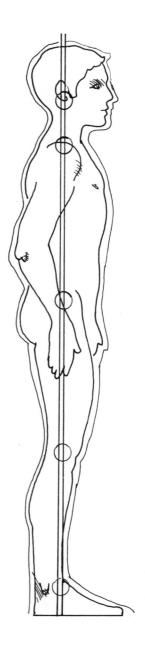

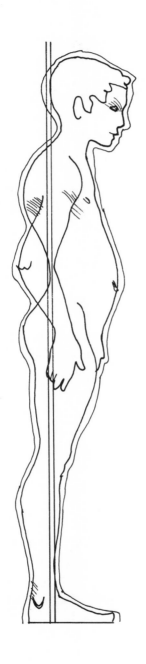

FIGURE 53.
Poor body alignment means that the head is too far forward, the ribs are cramped, and body weight is thrown in front of the knees while they are held backward. In this type of alignment, body weight is thrown on the ligaments instead of the bone structure that is designed to carry the weight.

your appearance. It projects youth, alertness, and confidence.

Actors do not confine age imagery to face make-up. Their most effective way of conveying aging is through posture—hunched over shoulders, drooping head, and a rounded back. The young actor carries his head high, even though he may be trembling inside with lack of confidence and fear of failure, and he camouflages the inner fear with an erect, confident-looking posture. A former actress with this youthful posture strode boldly onto the stage and happily announced with vigor that she was a 78-year-old grandmother—Gloria Swanson. No granny shoulders and rounded back for her.

A turkey neck, a widow's hump, and a bent back are all correctible.

"But I am so tall," one female university student complained. That is not a valid excuse, especially for the young. Six-foot-tall Rosalind Russell, the late well-known actress, was much admired for her beauty, even late into her life, when she was plagued with illness. Her proud, erect head and neck were very visible at the last luncheon she attended, when she addressed the crowd with the bearing of a Rose Queen. Even in these late years, her erect posture still gave the illusion of youth.

How can you tell if your head is straight? For the initial test, try the following. Go to a wall and place the back of your head, your shoulders, and your hips flat against the wall. Your heels should be two inches away from the wall, and your arms should be at your sides.

Your body is now aligned perfectly. That means that all your body parts are in line so that the body weight falls onto the bone structure, which is meant to bear weight. By touching the three crucial points —the back of your head, your shoulders, and the back of your hips—against the wall, you have achieved perfect posture. If you walk away from the wall and try to maintain the position of the body, however, you may feel odd, uncomfortable, or strained. These are all words used by people who were placing their body segments in perfect alignment for the first time in many years. Yet there is a very good reason for reporting that perfect posture feels odd or strained.

If, over the years, one has allowed his head to drop, his shoulders to cup, and his back to stoop, the body bindings in those areas will have shortened from dropping forward, and they will "protest" when forced to yield or lengthen in the new, straight position. Elongation demands have to be made gradually and practiced. Only when the bindings are stretched out to a more comfortable length will a person be able to hold his head tall, his neck long, and his shoulders square and feel perfectly comfortable and easy in a good posture position.

If you stretch your bindings, you not only will be growing more youthful as you grow older; you will be growing healthier and this could be correctly called "aging with a future."

During the late fifties and early sixties, because of the enormous popularity of Marilyn Monroe, it was very fashionable among teenagers to stand with their hips protruding excessively. If that position was maintained over many years without counteracting stretches, the body bindings that pass in front of the hips would become excessively shortened. If this shortening is maintained, it becomes mechanically impossible to place his hips where they belong, directly under the spine (see Figure 54).

The same problem exists for the individual who virtually "sits on his hips." There the bindings become shortened in the back part of the hips. In either case, the hips no longer swing easily; they are tightened, fixed, and stiff, and because of gravity, the weight of the body falls either too far front or too far to the rear when the person walks. The weight is thrown off the weight-bearing structures, namely the bones and joints, and the future health of those body parts is in danger (see Figure 55). By putting the power of positive stretching to use, you will serve a double purpose: you will make possible the correction of bad body alignment and you will be able to move body parts with comfort and ease, not strain and pain. The variety of head and neck stretches offered in this book is totally unnecessary to get the job of elongation done. The basic stretches outlined in Chapter 5 are sufficient. But people, being people, need many roads to Rome. Whichever road you choose, the objective—attaining the proper head and shoulder position in good posture for good body functioning—is the same (see Figure 56).

Although body freedom is necessary to align the body parts comfortably, a good way to test your posture is the old practice of placing a book on top of your head while standing with your hips, shoulders and the back of your head against the wall. Then, with the book balanced on your head, walk to the other side of the room and back to the wall. If the book is still on your head, you have maintained an erect position. This should give you an idea of what is meant by "straight," and it will help to develop erect posture (see Figure 57–59).

When traveling in the Orient, the absence of Western furniture frequently brings moans and groans from Westerners forced to sit on cushions or floors. So the relation of furniture to good body mechanics naturally comes to mind. Sitting badly can be harmful if protracted over many years. In the very best position, the feet should rest comfortably on the floor, and the ankles, knees, and hips should be at right angles. The back of the hips should touch the back of the chair or be supported in some way. The head should be up, and the chin should be level (see Figure 60). Pregnant women have found that sitting in a hard chair in this position is most restful over a period of time. Low, deep couches or seats look much more seductive, but curved and twisted spines will eventually complain if a person sits in them too long or habitually.

The person who works in a sitting position also has better posture when seated in a hard-back chair. One should lean forward from the hips, not the waist. This prevents rounded shoulders. The forearms should rest easily on the desk surface for support and balance (Figures 61 and 62).

While on the subject of furniture, the following suggestions are useful in arranging furniture. These were compiled over the years for patients who lived alone and had to move very cautiously in order to manage with leg or body injuries. They are general enough, however, to be useful to those who are healthy.

- Overstuffed chairs are hard to get out of. Although people who are very flexible, strong, and whose bindings are fully elongated can rise without difficulty, the inactive and the stiff cannot. Hard chairs with straight, supportive backs are best for long periods of sitting, and the back of the hips should touch the back of the chair.
- All clutter and knick-knacks are hazardous to indoor mobility, unless they are kept out of the main line of traffic. Extra end tables, lamps, and plants scattered throughout prevent brisk, clear walking in the home.
- Loose rugs are extremely dangerous for anyone, injured or not. The elderly report many hazards from this common source, especially in the dark. All rugs should be stationary and firmly fastened down.
- In the bedroom, the passageway between the bed and the bathroom should be clear and easy to travel. Intervening objects—wires, connections, or anything that could cause tripping—should be removed. The area should also be well lighted.
- A firm bed is most important for good posture. It is probably years since most people have tested their mattresses for firmness. A simple board between the mattress and springs will do much to firm up the bed. A flat pillow will help neck and shoulder bindings maintain their yield. All this should be taken care of before one gets old and has to prop up his or her body with numerous pillows to support the spine when faulty body mechanics have been allowed to persist.

So much for standing and sitting posture. What about posture while walking?

"Will the real Henri LM stand up?" Three elderly gentlemen, two of whom were impersonating the daredevil high diver, strode to their seats. Each one walked differently. One had a stiff gait, a heavy strutting. The second swung easily from the hips, pushing off from the ball of the foot. The third had a slight heel drag. Who was the high diver? The panel had to guess, and there could be only one at the age of 73. If his body was not free and flexible to adjust to the slightest change in motion as he came off the high dive—125 feet—he would have been severely injured as he hit the water and would have been dead long ago. It takes agility to shift weight and swing forward from the ball of your foot; you must be able to transfer weight easily, and this requires stretching.

I guessed that the high diver was the one who walked with relaxed knees and pushed off from the ball of the foot. Imagine my consternation if I was wrong! But I wasn't. The second gentlemen was the high-diving Henri, and his walk had told me his body was free. The other two had a rather typical gait for 73, which could have been corrected with some stretching.

For everyday practice, even without stretches, the following suggestions may be helpful:

- When standing for long periods, shift your weight from one leg to the other. This relieves undue strain on one set of joint bindings.
- Hard steps that practically punch holes in the sidewalk when you walk take more energy than an easy bounce and "soft" knees.

- Tuck your buttocks well under your spine when bending.
- Push up straight with your knees when returning to an erect position. This keeps your center of gravity close to the center of your body and saves energy.
- If you tend to drop your head and back when walking, try wearing a wide belt that fits snugly around your waist. This support will help the upper portion of your back stay erect and saves body energy.
- Change heel heights several times a day. This shift of balance will help maintain the flexibility of your heel cord, and there will be less chance for the Achilles tendon to become stiff and fixed.

Good, dynamic posture is based upon freedom of body parts, and that freedom brings lightness and joy in movement rather than the drag that so often comes with stiffness.

When we are young, we have wonderful elasticity. All it takes is an instinctive reminder, a little effort, and some excitement at new learning to regain our dynamic posture.

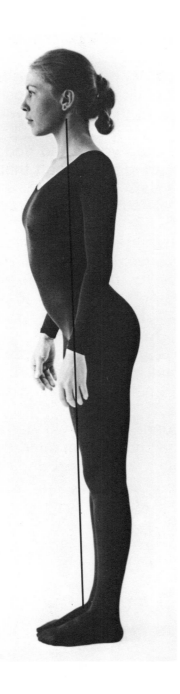

FIGURE 54.
Sway back posture causes weight to fall on the front of the hips and the ankles. At no point do the bones or joints share the weight.

FIGURE 55.
Sitting on the hip posture
causes weight to fall on
the back of the hips, knees,
and ankles. The bones and
joints do not help carry
the load.

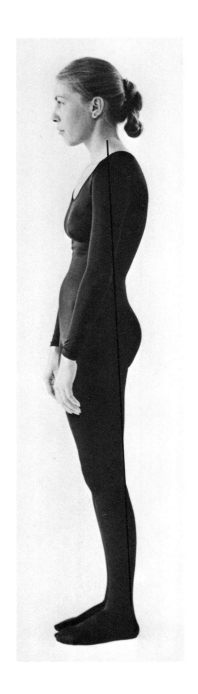

150

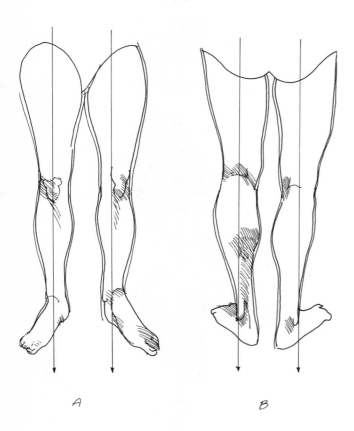

FIGURE 56.
When the bones and joints
do not bear the weight, it
falls on the soft tissues.
The arches and the sides
of the feet carry the burden
instead of the heel.

A   B

151

FIGURE 57.
The use of a posture screen is an excellent way to check body alignment. Are the shoulders and hips even? The screen is a simple device consisting of a frame approximately six feet tall and four feet wide, covered with strings about one inch apart that form a grid.

The hips of the same model, however, are perfectly straight (b).

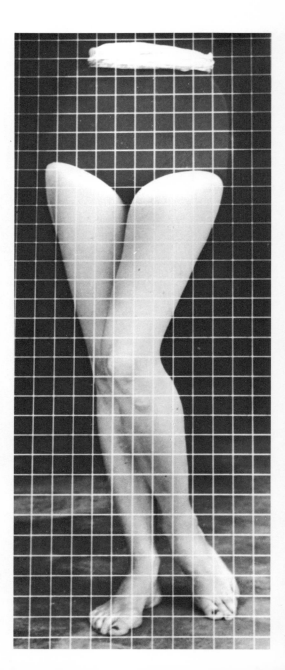

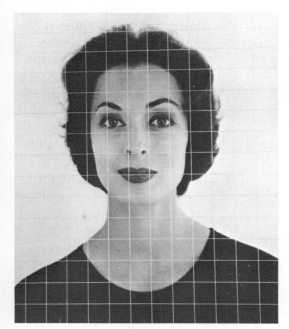

Here, the model's right shoulder is slightly lower than her left (a). This can come from always carrying bundles, books, and packages on the right side. It is most common in growing boys and girls and can be corrected.

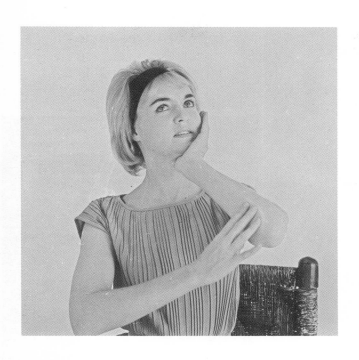

FIGURE 58.
Here are two variations of the neck stretch in Chapter 5.

In a comfortable seated position, place your chin in your right palm. Turn your head to the right and when you have gone as far as you can, give your right elbow a push beyond the stopping point. Be firm. Release slowly. Repeat on the opposite side. Be sure to release slowly between each stretch. Stretch three times on each side

An added force can be applied in the simple chin to chest stretch for releasing the bindings in the back of the neck. When your chin is as far down on your chest as possible, make a cradle with your arms and pull your head farther down with them. Concentrate on surrendering the back of your neck, saying all the time, "Let go, let go." Slowly come up straight. Stretch three times

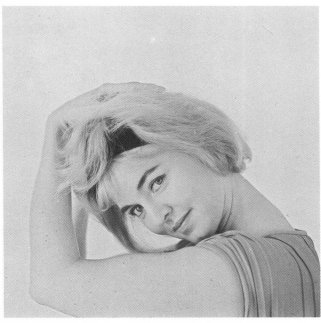

153

FIGURE 59.
A simple neck stretch can be done in the morning even before rising. Use the edge of your bed and lower your head over the edge. Allow it to hang for a count of 3. Then lift it slowly and hold for another count of 3. Repeat 5 times. Be sure to get the feeling of releasing at each stretch. When your head is hanging, concentrate on letting go, and when your chin is forward on your chest, concentrate on releasing the back of your neck. As always, to get the full benefit of the stretch, you must *release.*

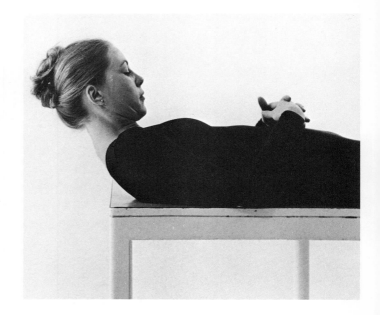

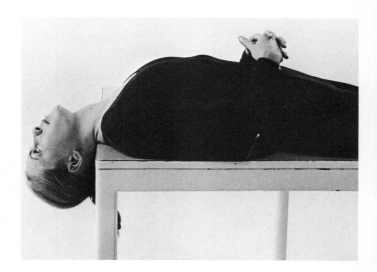

154

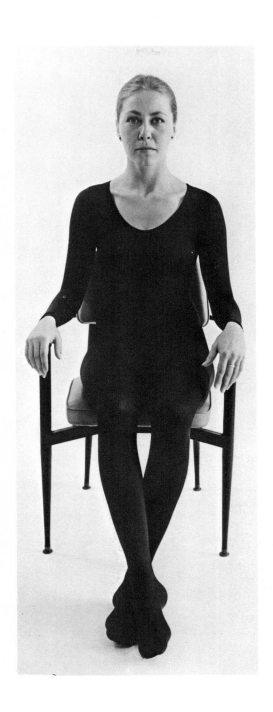

FIGURE 60.
Seated in a straight-back chair, cross your legs at the ankles. This is not only graceful, but it allows better circulation than crossing your legs at the knees.

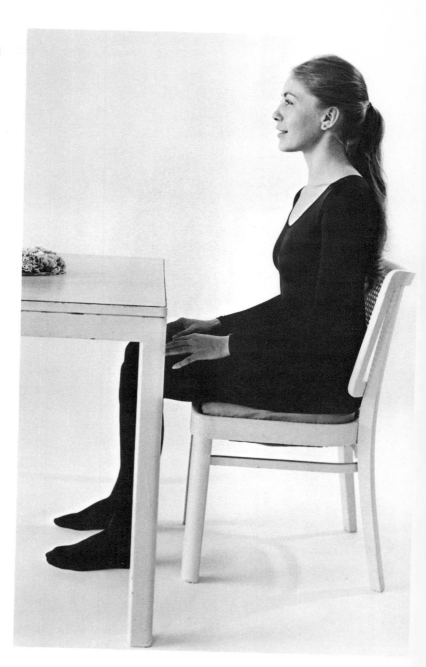

FIGURE 61.
Good Posture: Sitting
Position

156

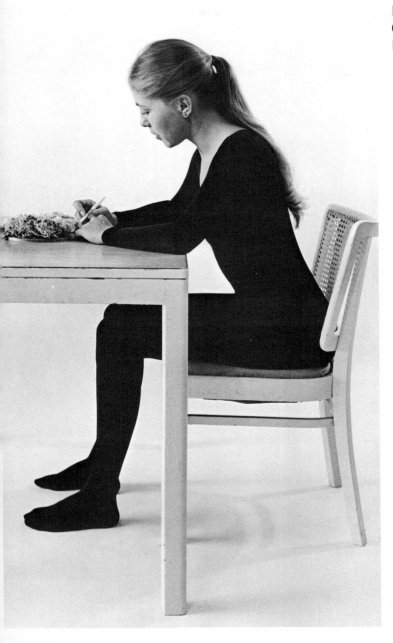

FIGURE 62.
Good Posture: Working
Position

157

11 One for The Road— Two for Buddies

Good
Health

One coronary attack or a single accident will create an immediate convert to healthy living where a dozen books and lectures fail. Picture yourself sliding down an escape chute from a wrecked airplane. You are alive! But are you healthy? The many months it takes for broken bones, torn ligaments, and bruised tissues to heal are witness to the hard fact most people's body parts have been inactive and stiff for many, many years. After a crash, the average 50-year-old has to learn to move all over again. As an orthopedist stated recently, "I can give you a new joint, but the use of the leg is up to you."

You must move for strength and stretch for range of motion, but even more has to take place for repair of damage and/or continuation of function. It is cardiac patients, injured patients, and sedentary middle-aged people to whom I owe a debt of gratitude. They have demonstrated the irrefutable truth —that to maintain normal range of motion at all body junctures is a safety factor, protection from injury, and insurance toward good health in the middle and later years.

Doing the three basic stretches daily can help one achieve good health, but what about the person who frankly states that he has not the time or, even more important, the inclination to exercise? Can anything be offered him that is beneficial?

"I hate exercise." This was how I was greeted one day by a prospective client whose medical doctor had prescribed activity. It took gentle persuasion and a demonstration that what he was about to learn was not exercising in the ordinary sense—that he could actually perform the movements while in bed—before he would agree to try them. He did not object to "resting" exercises.

His colleague, however, a musician who traveled a lot, was not so obstinate. He was willing to work standing up but wanted an extremely shortened routine. "What can I do in one exercise that will take care of the problem? I don't like to learn a routine because I will forget it."

Here was a new challenge—to find one meaningful stretch that would take care of several functions. More than anything else, the sedentary musician needed circulation stimulation. Expanding the folded-over areas in a cramped position was also necessary. In addition, range of motion would have to be restored and, lastly, he needed physical activity productive enough to take care of releasing tension from performing and traveling.

A former world-famous pianist, Oscar Levant, was often observed before concert performances pacing nervously back and forth behind the auditorium. He would chain-smoke and pound the pavement stiffly before curtain time. He too hated physical routines, and premature death eventually claimed him.

After trying many different single movements to achieve the goals of better circulation, improved relaxation, and stretching of many body junctures to full range, we introduced the stretch shown in Figure 63.

In order for it to do any good, every detail of it has to be done correctly. If you feel tingles, revitalization, and general exhilaration after doing six of these stretches (three on each side) three times daily, you are doing it correctly. Just three stretches to each side three times a day gives 18 instant body conditioners each day. This amounts to 540 stretches a month—not an inconsiderable amount of healthful movement.

Now that you have learned that one stretch a day can be beneficial in spite of its brevity, will you be able to discipline yourself or commit yourself to the daily repetition that it takes to get the desired results? In other words, can you do it alone each day? Some persons are able to achieve this readily. But what about the rest of the population?

A lot of people are not geared to working alone. They may start but then find it impossible to stick to it; yet if they have a companion or partner, they find it fun. Well, there is no rule that you must stretch alone. If you like companionship, find a partner; you can stretch together and check up on each other.

Test your ranges of motion as outlined in Chapter 3, and record the results. Make notes and keep track of each other.

When you have each determined where you are the tightest and where you have complete body freedom, help one another choose the special stretches that will benefit your body most. Start with the one that you need the most. The three basic stretches will cover it all, but you may prefer the resting routine or the highly active program. There are also variations with a knee push (see Figure 64) or a towel pull (see Figure 65), and a rib stretch for two (see Figure 66). Take your pick. Go through the whole repertoire if you are in a hurry to make corrections.

So what is involved in using the power of positive stretching? What are we actually dealing with? The instinctive ability to stretch is present in all of us and the techniques to put it into operation and maintain it are so simple it is almost hard to believe that we can benefit our bodies so much with so little.

The habit of brushing our teeth and grooming ourselves daily was inculcated in all of us not through individual choice, understanding, or personal striving for improvement. It was drilled there at an early age by our parents and teachers, who hoped that one day we would realize that our health and appearance depended upon the care and treatment of those body parts. If the power of stretching and the implementation of movement to keep us healthy and alert had been taught to us as children, how fortunate we would be as adults! It would feel different and unhealthy if we omitted it. (Have you ever skipped brushing your teeth for a day or two? Remember how unkept and unattractive you felt?)

For a final word, there are truths about life that contradict some common myths. New learning *is* possible as we go on in life. Physical impairment is not inevitable; it is directly related to habit. It is hard to change what we have repeated for 30 years or even for 30 days unless we use the 30 days to offset the many years of habitual behavior. That is not an impossible assignment. It just takes concentration of effort and repetition of the new to counteract the old.

An individual program where you can measure your progress at your own pace has a greater chance of succeeding than one that calls for competition, and it should appeal to those who feel that they can no longer compete. Improvement should be the only goal for everyone.

FIGURE 63.

Stand and point your right leg hard, making sure that you can feel the stretch all the way to your toes. At the same time, stretch your left arm high in the air until you can feel the stretch in your fingers. Point your chin toward the fingers of your left hand and s–t–r–e–t–c–h. Release slowly.

Remain standing and slump forward, bending your knees, dropping your head, and letting your arms fall loosely. Surrender completely; then straighten up.

Point your left leg hard, making sure that you feel the stretch in your toes. At the same time, stretch your right arm high in the air until you can feel the stretch in your fingers. Point your chin toward the fingers of your right hand and s–t–r–e–t–c–h. Release slowly. Slump forward again and let go. Repeat, alternating sides. Do three stretches on each side three times a day.

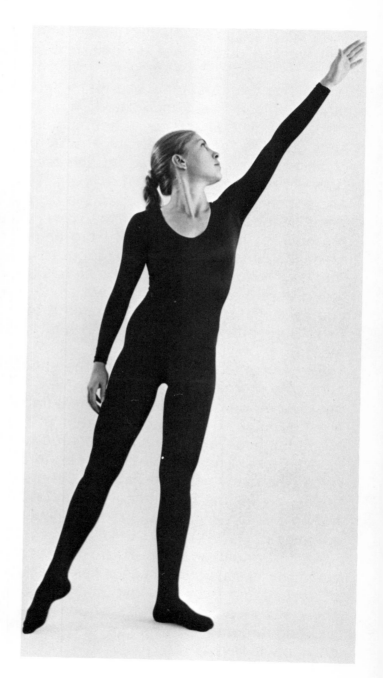

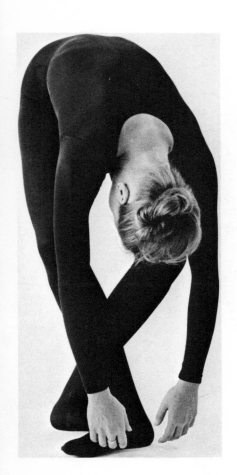

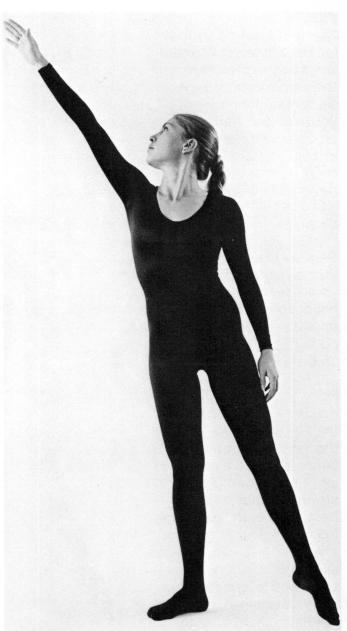

FIGURE 64.
The man in (a) discovered much tightness in the hip and knee region. His female partner, however, was completely mobile in this area. Her body bindings allowed her leg to lie flat on the floor (b). His did not.

Together they elongated their hip, knee, and ankle bindings. She placed a towel on the ball of her foot and gave a decided pull—in her case to maintain flexibility. He placed his hand firmly at the ball of the foot and strongly forced the knee down into a straight position or as close to one as possible (c).

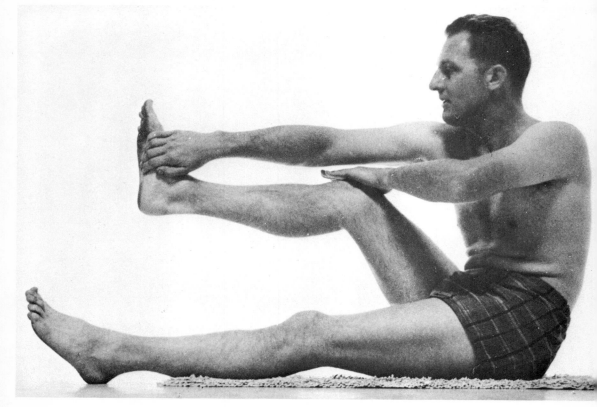

(a)

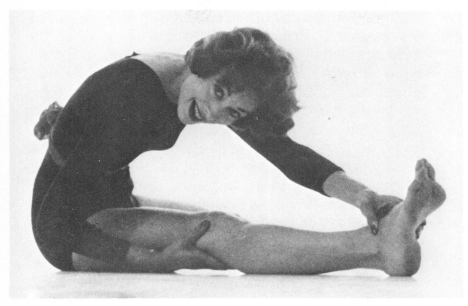

(b)

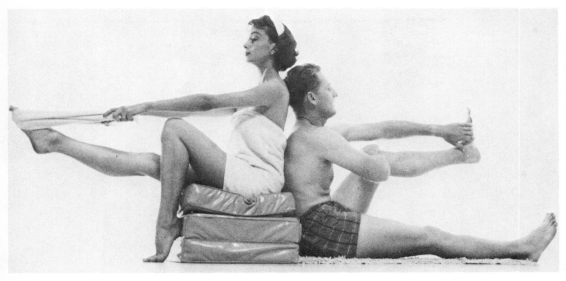

(c)

167

Good Health

Since the loss of mobility and the subsequent effort of getting around tends to isolate anyone, it is most crucial and desirable to maintain one's mobility in order to remain involved with other people. Since the majority of our population retains fairly good health up to 60 years of age, any program, even a minimal one, as detailed in Chapter 6, can prolong mobility and, consequently, promote better health. It is never too late to try to improve, and because it hurts to be a "big stiff," most people will surely show some improvement.

One last note: heart fitness is essential for living, so any program that helps the heart and blood vessels to better health has priority over any other, but (and this is of priority in its own right) the good health of your body bindings is essential to feeling well. And when you feel well, other good things are within your grasp, particularly the ability to make someone else happy too.

FIGURE 65.
The leg and knee bindings
can also be stretched by a
towel pulled around the
ball of the foot.

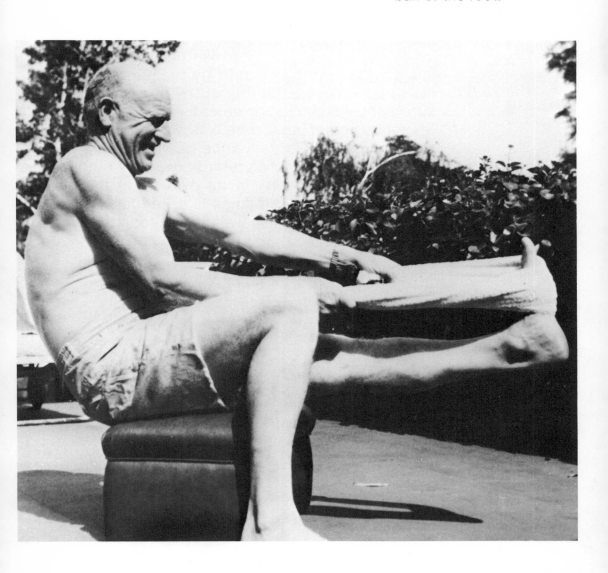

FIGURE 66.
Another stretch for two is fun and elongates the rib cage. Sit back to back, raise your arms overhead, and clasp hands. Slowly and gently, one partner should lean forward, pulling the other over with him as far as possible. Then alternate sides. It is a challenge to see how far you can increase the arc of the stretch.

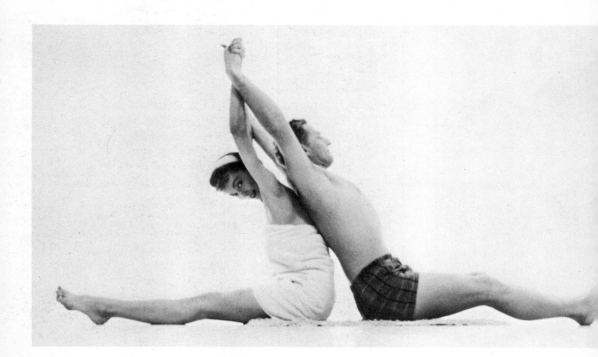

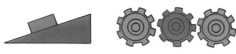

USBORNE UNDERSTANDING SCIENCE
MACHINES

Clive Gifford

Consultant: **Dr. Bryson Gore**

Designed by **John Barker**

Illustrated by **Andy Burton**

Additional illustration by **Kevin Lyles**

Additional designs:
John Russell, Steve Wright and **Steve Page**

Series Editor: **Jane Chisholm**

Technical Advisor:
L.F.E. Coombs

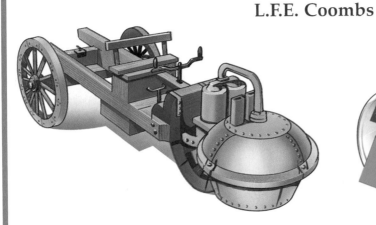

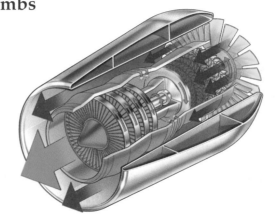

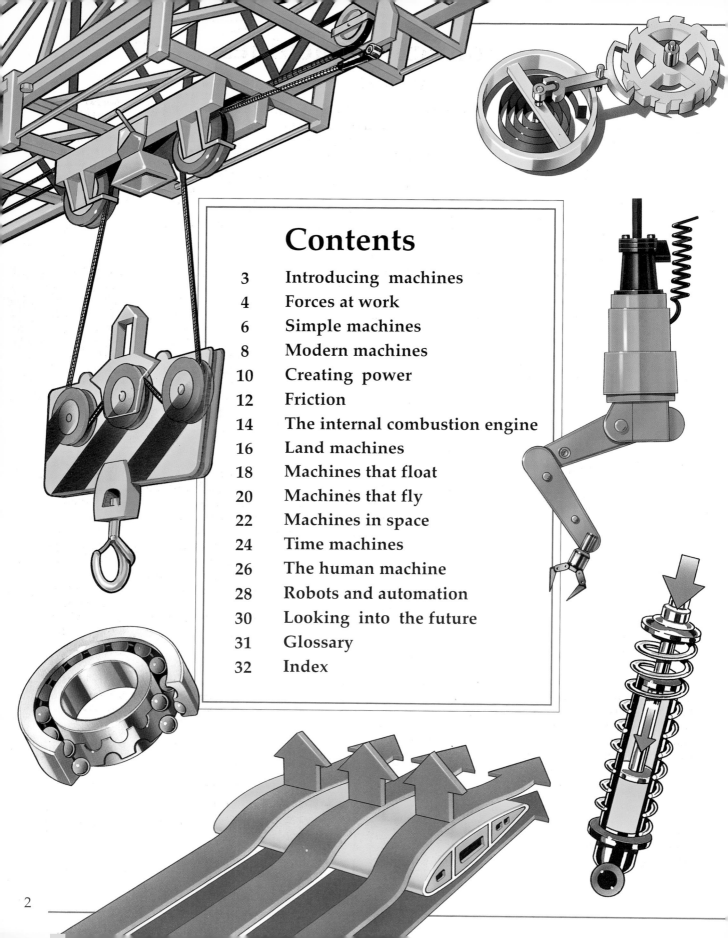

Contents

Introducing machines

You may think of a machine as something very powerful and complicated, like a crane, a car engine or an aircraft, but a simple stone axe and a pair of scissors are machines as well. Scientists describe a machine as any device which makes work easier, or increases the speed at which it is done. The word comes from the Ancient Greek *mechos*, which means "to help make things easy".

There are many hundreds of different machines all around you, from tweezers to trains, from bottle-openers to bulldozers.

A hand drill is a machine powered by turning its handle.

Mechanics

The rules and principles which govern how machines, or parts of machines, move are grouped together into an area of science called mechanics.

Many machines today, such as pocket calculators and washing machines, do not rely solely on mechanical action in order to work. This is because they are powered by electricity, or controlled by electronics. This book concentrates on the mechanical aspects of machines, whether or not they use electricity.

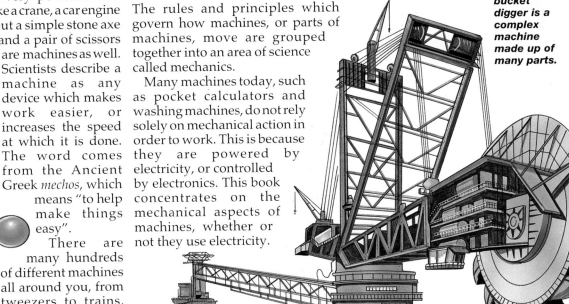

This huge bucket digger is a complex machine made up of many parts.

What machines do

What all machines have in common, from the simplest to the most complicated, is that they exert some kind of action on an object. This action is called a force.

A force is any sort of pushing or pulling action. For example, a crane pulls a load off the ground, while a bulldozer pushes earth out of the way. You can't see a force, but you can often feel it, or see it in action. For example, when you are outdoors, you can feel the force of a strong wind pushing against you. When you are indoors, you can't feel the wind's force, but you can watch the way it blows the leaves around. In both cases, you can't actually see the force, but you can see its effect.

How machines help

Machines make your life easier in many ways. Some machines help make jobs quicker. For example, a car can help you travel a long distance many times faster than if you were walking.

Some machines allow you to do a job with much less effort. A spade can dig a large hole a lot easier than if you just used your bare hands.

Some machines can do a better job than you could do on your own. A nutcracker breaks the shell of a nut, without smashing the nut itself. Other machines do more than just help; they perform jobs that we could not do by ourselves at all. Many transport machines fall into this category. Although we cannot fly by ourselves, we can do so in a machine called an aircraft.

Some machines can work in places where people cannot. This Viking I Spacecraft visited Mars and took photographs there.

Words in *italic* type

Words which appear in *italic* type and are followed by a small star (for example, *compound machine**) can be found in the glossary on page 31, together with other important terms relating to machines.

Forces at work

All machines - from the simplest screwdriver to the most complex spacecraft - have one thing in common: they deal with forces. What a machine does is to take a force and change its size or direction.

In most situations, an object has several forces acting upon it, usually from different directions. When an object is still, all the opposing forces are balanced. For something to move, the force in one direction has to be greater than the force in the other. For example, a tug of war will be won by the team that pulls the hardest. When both teams are pulling as hard as each other, there is no movement because the opposing forces are balanced.

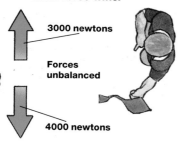

The team pulling with the most force wins.

3000 newtons

Forces unbalanced

4000 newtons

Forces are measured in newtons, named after the British scientist, Sir Isaac Newton (1642-1727).

Different types of forces

There are two different types of forces: turning, or rotary, forces, which move in a circle; and linear forces, which move in a straight line. Many machines are designed to convert one type of force to another. For example, the force of an aircraft propeller turning around quickly pulls the aircraft forward.

Work, energy and power

Scientists use the term "work" to mean the amount of force applied, multiplied by the distance over which the force is maintained. Work describes how much effort is used and is measured in joules. Work is only done when something is moved.

Work = Force x Distance (in meters (3.25ft)).

This person is pushing a box with a force of 100 newtons for a distance of 3m.

3 x 100 = 300

The man has performed 300 joules of work.

"Power" is the rate at which work is done. In the past it was measured in horsepower, but now it is measured in watts, named after the steam engineer, James Watt (1736-1819). Power is calculated with the following equation:

$$Power = \frac{Work\ (in\ joules)}{Time\ (in\ seconds)}\ watts$$

For example, if the person in the diagram above had done the job in one minute, the average power would have equalled 5 watts.

$$\frac{300\ joules}{60\ seconds} = 5\ watts$$

"Energy" is the ability to do work. Like work, it is measured in joules. There are many kinds of energy: heat, light, chemical, mechanical, nuclear and kinetic energy (the energy of movement). The heavier something is and the faster it moves, the more kinetic energy it possesses.

A number of actions can convert energy from one type to another. For example, the kinetic energy of rubbing two sticks together can change into heat energy which may eventually set the sticks on fire. Sometimes one energy type can be converted into several different forms. For example, when a light is switched on, electrical energy is supplied to a light bulb, releasing light and heat energy.

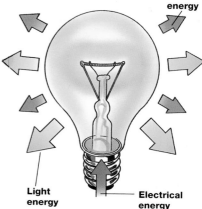

Heat energy

Light energy

Electrical energy

Losing energy

All machines waste energy; they convert some of it into forms they cannot use. The energy efficiency of a machine is a measure of how good it is at converting energy into the forms that it does want and can use. For example, a buckled bicycle wheel is less efficient than a new one. As the buckled wheel scrapes against the side of the cycle frame, it turns some of its forward movement into *friction**. The scraping sound you hear, as the wheel rubs against the frame, is more energy being wasted as it is converted into sound energy.

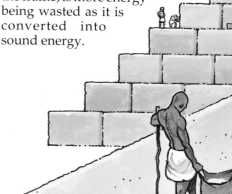

4

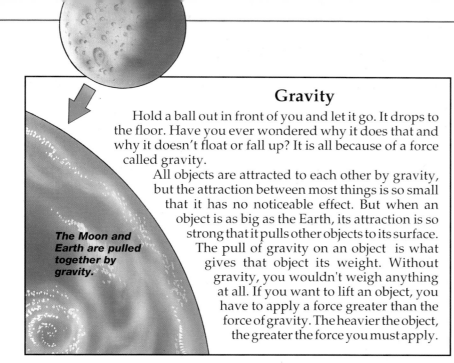

Gravity

Hold a ball out in front of you and let it go. It drops to the floor. Have you ever wondered why it does that and why it doesn't float or fall up? It is all because of a force called gravity.

All objects are attracted to each other by gravity, but the attraction between most things is so small that it has no noticeable effect. But when an object is as big as the Earth, its attraction is so strong that it pulls other objects to its surface.

The pull of gravity on an object is what gives that object its weight. Without gravity, you wouldn't weigh anything at all. If you want to lift an object, you have to apply a force greater than the force of gravity. The heavier the object, the greater the force you must apply.

The Moon and Earth are pulled together by gravity.

Inclined planes

The Ancient Egyptians built huge stone structures called pyramids, the largest of which was some 146m (480ft) high. That's as tall as 90 people standing on each other's shoulders. The large rocks used for making these structures were lifted using a slope called an inclined plane, or ramp.

Lifting a rock straight up requires a lot of force over a short distance. A gentle slope means that the force is applied over a much greater distance, but the force needed is reduced to well within human capacity. The amount of work that goes into lifting an object cannot be altered, but the inclined plane changes the way the work is actually done.

The work needed to lift the rock a specific height is equal to the force multiplied by the distance over which you apply that force. By increasing the distance, you can reduce the amount of force required. In the example below, a load travels eight times as far up a slope as it would if it had been lifted straight up. But it only requires an eighth of the force to lift it.

8 times the distance = 1/8th of the force needed

Slope distance: 80m (260ft)

Vertical distance: 10m (32.5ft)

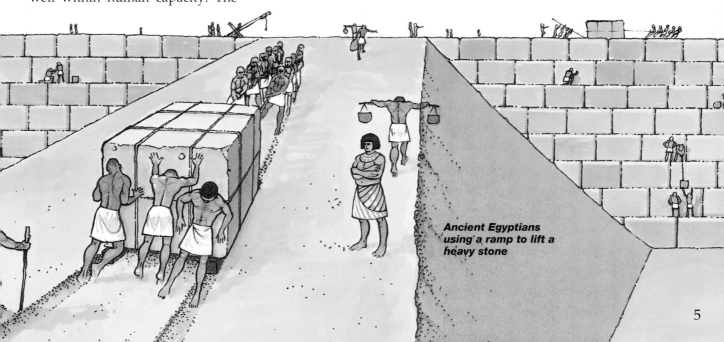

Ancient Egyptians using a ramp to lift a heavy stone

Simple machines

The most basic machine, which is called a "simple machine", is one that is made from very few parts and only alters a single force. It may modify the type of force (for example, by turning a straight line force into a turning one), or it may alter the direction, size or strength of the force. Some of the most important ones have been in use for well over 2000 years.

The 2nd century Greek scientist, Hero of Alexandria, believed that even the most complex machines were in fact made up of five simple ones: the inclined plane, the pulley, the screw, the lever and the wheel. The inclined plane was looked at on page 5. These two pages look at the other four.

A tower crane uses a combination of levers and pulleys to lift heavy weights.

Levers

A lever is a straight rod which revolves around a fixed point, called a fulcrum or pivot. It is used to change the size of a turning force. The object being moved by the lever is called the load and the force applied is called the effort.

A lever with the load and effort an equal distance from, but on opposite sides of, the pivot point can be used as a weighing balance. The object being weighed is the load and the weights used to equal the load provide the effort.

A simple balance

This pole is the lever.

Pivot

Load

Effort

Increasing force and distance

A lever can be used to increase the force applied. A lever with the pivot point closer to the load than the effort will produce a strong force over a short distance. A crowbar and a spade are both examples of force-increasing levers.

A lever with the pivot point closer to the effort produces a weaker force, but one which works over a greater distance. Fishing rods and hammers are both examples of distance-increasing levers.

These heavy blocks are called counterweights. They are used to balance the jib.

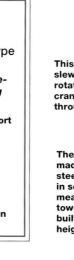

These thick wires help strengthen the jib. They are called cantilever cables.

Cranes like this can be as high as 200m (630ft).

Crane driver's cab

This is the slewing gear. It rotates the crane's jib through 360°.

The tower is made of strong steel and comes in sections. This means that the tower can be built to any height.

Making two levers

You can easily make both types of levers with a short ruler and a pencil. The distance between the effort and pivot points will determine which type of lever it is.

A force-increasing lever

Ruler lifts book.

Load

Pencil acts as the pivot point.

Long distance between effort and pivot points

Effort

Ball of paper flies into air.

A distance-increasing lever

Effort

Short distance between effort and pivot points

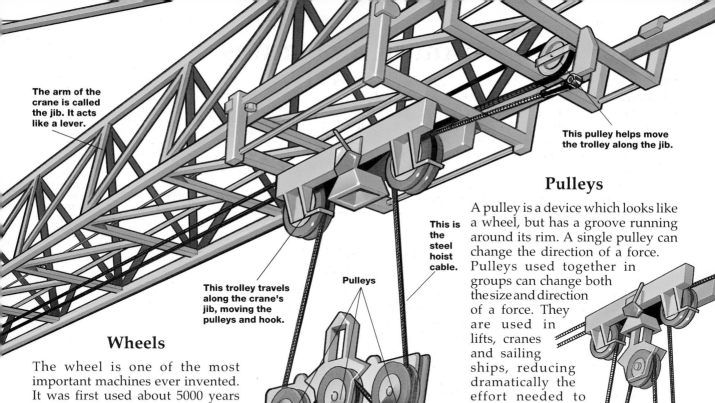

The arm of the crane is called the jib. It acts like a lever.

This pulley helps move the trolley along the jib.

This trolley travels along the crane's jib, moving the pulleys and hook.

This is the steel hoist cable.

Pulleys

The hoist mechanism

Pulleys greatly increase the load that the crane can lift.

Pulleys

A pulley is a device which looks like a wheel, but has a groove running around its rim. A single pulley can change the direction of a force. Pulleys used together in groups can change both the size and direction of a force. They are used in lifts, cranes and sailing ships, reducing dramatically the effort needed to raise a load. The pulleys can be moved far apart. This greatly increases the distance the hoist cable travels, but reduces the force required to lift the load.

Pulley wheel

The hoist cable travels a greater distance with the pulleys apart.

Wheels

The wheel is one of the most important machines ever invented. It was first used about 5000 years ago in Mesopotamia, in an area now called Iraq, originally as a potter's wheel, and then as part of a simple cart. It forms the basis of many other devices such as gears (see page 8).

A solid wheel acts like a 360° lever which turns around a central fixed point, called an axle. When an axle is turned, the wheel turns with it. But because the wheel is much bigger than the axle, it covers a greater distance. The axle's circular motion is converted by the wheel into a straight line movement which can move loads across the ground.

A wheel can also be used to increase a force. If a wheel is turned, it moves a greater distance than the axle, but it turns the axle with more force. This is how a screwdriver works. Its handle is bigger than the bit, so that when the handle is turned the bit moves less far, but with greater force.

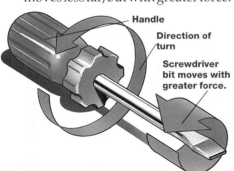

Handle

Direction of turn

Screwdriver bit moves with greater force.

Screws

A screw can change a turning force into a linear force along the direction of the screw's axle. For example, when a corkscrew is turned, it moves forward into the cork. One way to think of a screw is as an inclined plane wrapped around an axle. As the screw is turned, the axle is slowly pulled forward, carrying the screw with it.

A screw can also be used to change the size of a force. The angle of the thread spiralling along the axle acts like the angle of an inclined plane. It is called the pitch. The size of the pitch determines how far the screw moves forward as it is turned, and with what force. The greater the pitch, the more the screw moves forward. The greater the distance the screw moves, the smaller the force it moves with.

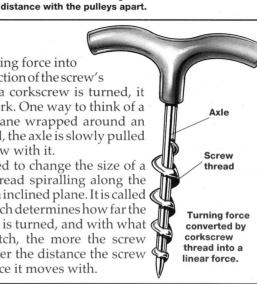

Axle

Screw thread

Turning force converted by corkscrew thread into a linear force.

Modern machines

Modern machines, such as robots and spaceships, have come a long way since the primitive lever. Advances have been made possible through the adaptation of older simple machines as well as the invention of new ones.

Hero of Alexandria (see page 6) believed that all machines could be made up from a combination of the five simple ones he had named. But 1500 years later, the great Italian scientist, inventor and artist, Leonardo da Vinci (1452-1519), listed as many as 22 simple machines in his book *Elements of Machines*.

Today's machines include even more simple machines (such as the airfoil), developments of simple machines (such as the gear) and complex machines, like the helicopter, which are made up of a large number of simple ones.

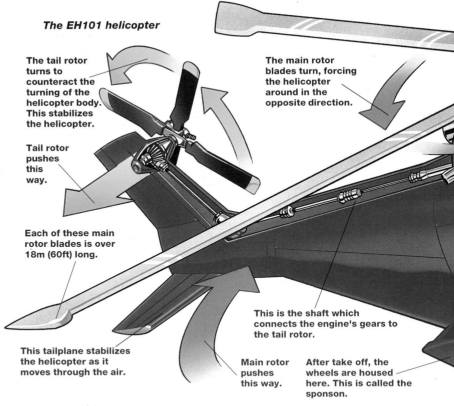

The EH101 helicopter

The tail rotor turns to counteract the turning of the helicopter body. This stabilizes the helicopter.

Tail rotor pushes this way.

Each of these main rotor blades is over 18m (60ft) long.

The main rotor blades turn, forcing the helicopter around in the opposite direction.

This is the shaft which connects the engine's gears to the tail rotor.

This tailplane stabilizes the helicopter as it moves through the air.

Main rotor pushes this way.

After take off, the wheels are housed here. This is called the sponson.

Gears

Gears are machines which can alter the size and direction of a turning force. Often they have grooves or teeth on their edges. This enables them to interlock with other gears without slipping. If two gears are positioned with their edges touching, turning one makes the other turn, but in the opposite direction. If you make the gears different sizes, the smaller one will turn faster, allowing the force to be applied over different distances.

Airfoils

The airfoil is a machine which, like the lever, is designed to lift things. Given its name by British engineer F.W. Lanchester in 1884, the airfoil has become extremely important in the modern world. Yacht sails and aircraft wings are just two things which owe their shape to the principle of the airfoil

When an airfoil-shaped wing moves through the air, its front or leading edge divides the air, forcing it under and over.

A cross section of an aircraft wing

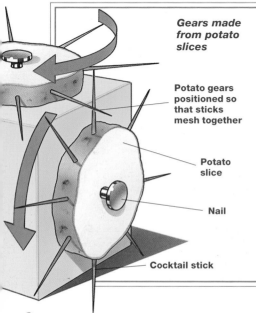

Gears made from potato slices

Potato gears positioned so that sticks mesh together

Potato slice

Nail

Cocktail stick

Making your own gears

You can make your own set of gears using potatoes. You will need two 1cm (½") thick round slices of raw potato, a shoebox, two nails and 16 cocktail sticks.

Push an equal number of sticks into the edges of the potato, spacing them at regular intervals. Using the nails, mount one of the gears on the side of the box, and the other on the bottom, with the cocktail sticks meshing. Hold the box up and turn the gear on the side of the box. You will find that the gear on the top of the box goes around at an angle of 90° to the side gear.

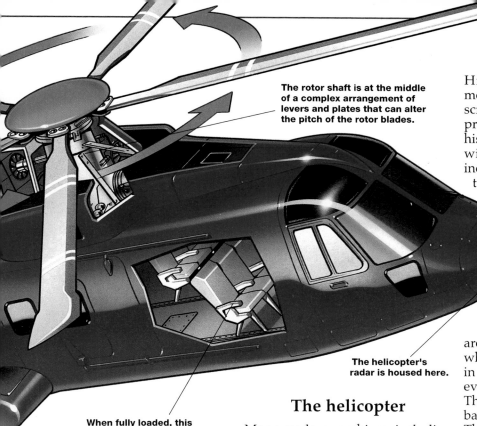

The rotor shaft is at the middle of a complex arrangement of levers and plates that can alter the pitch of the rotor blades.

The helicopter's radar is housed here.

When fully loaded, this helicopter weighs over 10,000kg (22,000lbs). It can carry up to 30 passengers or 16 stretcher patients.

His model used a clockwork mechanism to turn a short vertical screw, not unlike a modern ship's propeller. Scientists now know that his machine could not have worked without a number of advances, including the invention of the airfoil, the tail rotor and the internal combustion engine (see pages 14-15).

A modern helicopter is lifted into the air by a number of airfoils, called rotor blades. These are much more efficient than da Vinci's short screw.

When the main rotor blades are turning, they produce a force which wants to rotate the helicopter in the opposite direction (because every force has an opposite force). The helicopter needs something to balance the force of the main rotor. This is the job of the tail rotor.

The tail rotor stabilizes the helicopter, but also directs it left or right. Its thrust is normally balanced with that of the main rotor, to allow the craft to travel straight ahead. Decreasing the tail rotor's thrust lets the tail be pushed in the direction that the main rotor is turning. Increasing the thrust does the opposite.

The helicopter

Many modern machines, including helicopters, were actually first thought of centuries ago. But they could not be successfully built until new techniques and inventions had been pioneered. As far as we know, the first person to design a helicopter was Leonardo da Vinci.

Both the top and bottom surfaces of the airfoil are curved, but the curve on the top is steeper. This means that the air moving over the airfoil has more distance to go than the air moving under it. As a result, the air going over the top moves faster and its pressure (the force with which the air presses down on the wing) decreases. This means the pressure forcing the wing up is now stronger than the pressure forcing it down. This makes the wing rise.

A model of da Vinci's helicopter design

The wing lifts up.

Air travels over the wing.

Air travels under the wing.

Air is divided by the wing's front edge.

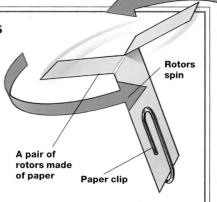

Make your own rotors

To make your own simple set of rotor blades, take a piece of paper 8cm x 2cm (3¼" x ¾"). Place a small paper clip on one end and make a tear of 3cm (1¼") at the other end. Bend the two flaps back, as shown here, and throw it into the air. After starting its fall, the two flaps should act as rotors, spinning the craft around as it descends.

Rotors spin

A pair of rotors made of paper

Paper clip

Creating power

All machines require some form of power to enable them to work. With some simple devices, such as a hammer or a cart, this comes from a person or an animal. But many machines require more power than an animal can provide. So special machines are designed with the sole purpose of providing it. One of the most up-to-date of these is the turbofan engine (shown on the right).

A turbofan engine is really two machines in one. A turbine engine powers a large fan at the front of the engine which sucks air through to produce thrust.

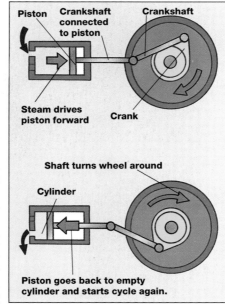

Water wheels and windmills

The earliest machines for power, such as the windmill and the water wheel, date back as much as 2000 years. They both use forms of power that come directly from nature.

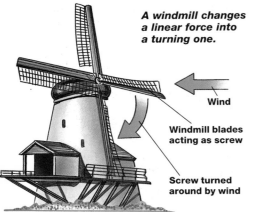

A windmill changes a linear force into a turning one.

Wind

Windmill blades acting as screw

Screw turned around by wind

A water wheel placed in the path of flowing water uses the movement of the water to turn the wheel. In other words, it converts the linear force of the water into a turning force. The power produced by water wheels was used to operate machines in early industries, such as weaving and woodworking.

A windmill acts like a screw facing into the wind. The moving air drives the windmill's sails around. Windmills were used for centuries to provide power to grind corn and pump water away from low-lying areas. They are still used in some places today for the same tasks. There are also many modern windmills, called wind generators, which are used to generate electricity.

The steam engine and how it works

For centuries, industries had to rely on power from windmills and water wheels. But these machines weren't always practical, as they were dependent on the weather to supply them with enough wind or water.

All this changed dramatically with the development of the steam engine at the end of the 17th century. Steam power lay at the heart of the Industrial Revolution of the 18th and 19th centuries. It revolutionized transport and made possible the growth of new industries, such as iron and steel.

Steam engines work by burning coal or oil to heat water, then turning heat energy into mechanical force. Water is boiled inside a sealed container, creating

Piston

Crankshaft connected to piston

Crankshaft

Steam drives piston forward

Crank

Shaft turns wheel around

Cylinder

Piston goes back to empty cylinder and starts cycle again.

steam. This has a much greater volume than water (about 2000 times as much) and so it expands. As it does this, it creates *pressure** which pushes a piston (a close-fitting metal rod) forward inside a tube called a cylinder.

The linear force of the piston is converted into a turning force by a device called a crank. A crank is a form of wheel which is joined to the piston by a connecting rod. As the piston moves to and fro, the crank turns, driving a machine's gears or wheels.

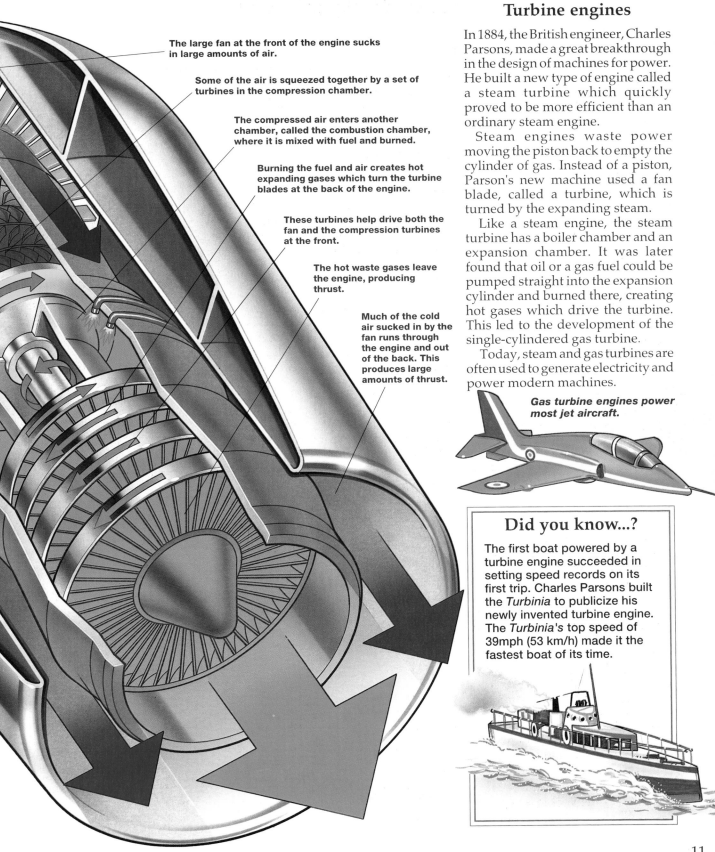

The large fan at the front of the engine sucks in large amounts of air.

Some of the air is squeezed together by a set of turbines in the compression chamber.

The compressed air enters another chamber, called the combustion chamber, where it is mixed with fuel and burned.

Burning the fuel and air creates hot expanding gases which turn the turbine blades at the back of the engine.

These turbines help drive both the fan and the compression turbines at the front.

The hot waste gases leave the engine, producing thrust.

Much of the cold air sucked in by the fan runs through the engine and out of the back. This produces large amounts of thrust.

Turbine engines

In 1884, the British engineer, Charles Parsons, made a great breakthrough in the design of machines for power. He built a new type of engine called a steam turbine which quickly proved to be more efficient than an ordinary steam engine.

Steam engines waste power moving the piston back to empty the cylinder of gas. Instead of a piston, Parson's new machine used a fan blade, called a turbine, which is turned by the expanding steam.

Like a steam engine, the steam turbine has a boiler chamber and an expansion chamber. It was later found that oil or a gas fuel could be pumped straight into the expansion cylinder and burned there, creating hot gases which drive the turbine. This led to the development of the single-cylindered gas turbine.

Today, steam and gas turbines are often used to generate electricity and power modern machines.

Gas turbine engines power most jet aircraft.

Did you know...?

The first boat powered by a turbine engine succeeded in setting speed records on its first trip. Charles Parsons built the *Turbinia* to publicize his newly invented turbine engine. The *Turbinia's* top speed of 39mph (53 km/h) made it the fastest boat of its time.

Friction

All machines are inefficient. This means that they waste power. One of the things that always wastes power is a force called friction.

Friction is the scientific name for the rubbing together of two or more things. You can feel the effects of friction if you rub your hands together. The tighter you press your hands, the greater the friction, and the greater the effort needed for them to slide over each other. As you rub them together, they warm up. If you kept rubbing them, the friction would create wear and your hands would develop blisters.

Friction wastes power, generates heat and creates wear. Reducing it can enable machines to move faster and with less effort. But friction can also be very useful. Without some friction between your foot and the ground, you would be slipping all the time. The soles of shoes are often designed to create extra friction, to give you more grip in slippery or muddy conditions.

Wedges in soles

Running shoes have wedges which dig into the ground, creating extra friction and grip.

Creating smooth surfaces

There are a number of ways of reducing friction. One way is to use a material which has a non-sticky surface, such as PTFE (a substance used as a covering on non-stick saucepans and on the moving parts of industrial machinery).

The second method of reducing friction is to place a thin layer of liquid between two moving surfaces. The liquid is much smoother than the surfaces and helps create less of the sticky movement which causes friction. Using liquids in this way is called lubrication. Oiling the wheels and handlebars of a bicycle is one example of lubrication.

Rolling friction

When two flat surfaces slide over each other, they rub and create friction. But if the sliding movement can be converted into a rolling movement, the friction can be reduced enormously.

Putting marbles under a book helps it move easily.

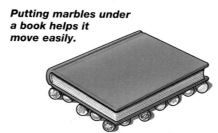

This is because a round surface constantly lifts off a flat surface, so that less of the time is spent with the two surfaces sliding over each other.

A ball bearing

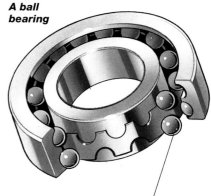

The area of contact between the balls and the moving parts is very small.

Ball bearings are an example of rolling friction used in many complex machines. They consist of one or several circles of steel balls, which separate two sliding surfaces. The balls are allowed to rotate freely within a track, called a ball race.

This thruster blasts a jet of air out. It can turn left and right and helps steer the craft.

These propellers push the craft forward.

This craft has four engines, two for the back propellers and two on the side to power the fans.

The fans suck air in to fill the skirt.

This air flows through holes in the bottom of the skirt underneath the craft.

The friction of air

A moving vehicle encounters friction, even from the air it moves through. To reduce air friction, vehicles are often designed with as smooth and sleek a shape as possible. This is described as streamlining and it helps create the smallest possible amount of resistance in air. New car models are put through *wind tunnel** tests to find which body shapes have the best streamlining.

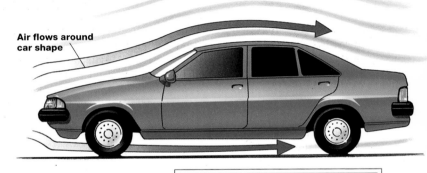

Air flows around car shape

Getting off the ground

Contact with air produces far less friction than contact with land or water. This is one of the reasons why aircraft can travel faster than boats, cars or trains. But some forms of land and sea transport are designed to reduce the friction they encounter by removing direct contact with the surface they travel over. Two examples of this are magnetic levitation trains (see page 30) and air-cushioned vehicles, known as ACVs.

An ACV uses a powerful cushion of air to lift itself off the ground. The body, or hull, of an ACV doesn't touch the surface it is moving over. This helps reduce friction and means that the craft can cross both water and solid ground.

This modern Air Cushioned Vehicle is a BHC AP.1-88. It can carry 101 passengers and has a top speed of 92km/h (56mph).

The skirt has been cut away to show how the ACV works.

How powerful is air?

The weight of air pressing down on the ground is called air pressure. This pressure can be concentrated to form a powerful force. For example, a pneumatic drill, powered by compressed air, can produce a force strong enough to power a special chisel to crack rock.

To see for yourself just how powerful air pressure can be, try lifting a heavy book up from the table with a paper bag. Place most of the bag under the book and then blow up the bag. The air in the bag will easily lift the book up.

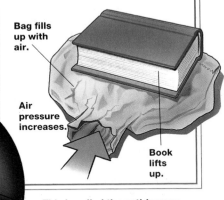

Bag fills up with air.

Air pressure increases.

Book lifts up.

This is called the anti-bounce web. It helps support the skirt.

Holes in the anti-bounce web allow air to pass into, but not out of, the outer chamber.

The outer chamber of the skirt is kept full of air. This makes the craft more stable in rough weather.

The air under the ACV lifts it up off the ground.

These flexible parts are called fingers. They help the ACV travel over rough surfaces, while trapping the air beneath the craft.

Some of the air escapes from the fingers as the craft travels over uneven surfaces.

The internal combustion engine

One of the most important inventions of modern times is the internal combustion engine. It is powerful and efficient for its relatively small size, and has been used to power many different machines, from lawn mowers and chain saws to cars and aircraft.

Developed in the late 19th century, the first internal combustion engine had a single cylinder and used an oil-based fuel called gasoline instead of coal. It was called an internal combustion engine because the fuel was burned or combusted inside the same chamber that contained the piston.

The combustion cycle

The process of burning fuel to create gases which expand and push the piston is called the combustion cycle. Each cycle involves a certain number of movements of the piston. Each upward or downward movement is called a stroke. Most modern internal combustion (IC) engines used in cars are called four-stroke engines. This is because the piston moves up twice and down twice in each cycle, making a total of four strokes. Once stroke four has been completed, the engine repeats the whole cycle. Below is a diagram of the four-stroke cycle.

The four-stroke combustion cycle

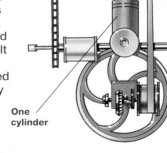
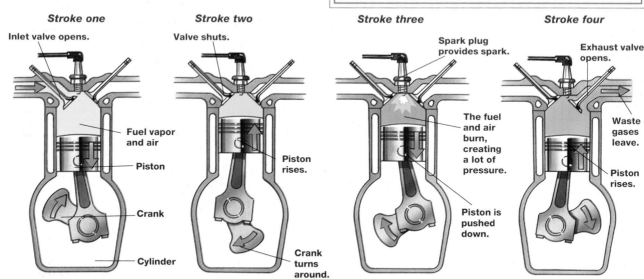

Stroke one

Inlet valve opens.

Fuel vapor and air

Piston

Crank

Cylinder

Stroke two

Valve shuts.

Piston rises.

Crank turns around.

Stroke three

Spark plug provides spark.

The fuel and air burn, creating a lot of pressure.

Piston is pushed down.

Stroke four

Exhaust valve opens.

Waste gases leave.

Piston rises.

During the first stroke of the combustion cycle, a valve, called the inlet valve, opens at the top of the cylinder. A mixture of fuel vapor and air is sucked in by the piston as it moves down the cylinder.

During the second stroke, the inlet valve shuts and the piston rises, squeezing the fuel and air mixture. This compression heats it up. As the piston reaches the top of its stroke, the mixture is ignited.

During the third stroke, the mixture burns rapidly, increasing its pressure. This pushes the piston down. It is this stroke that produces the power which can be used to drive other machines.

During the fourth stroke, another valve, called the exhaust valve, opens at the top of the cylinder. As the piston returns to the top of the cylinder, it pushes out the remains of the burned gases.

Powering wheels

Getting the power from an internal combustion engine to a vehicle's wheels is the job of a set of machines known as the transmission. The engine crankshaft is part of the transmission and runs straight from the engine. It is connected to a set of gears which greatly increase the maximum and minimum speeds at which the shaft can turn. This set of gears is called the gearbox.

The power is transmitted from the gearbox to the wheels, via a series of joints and shafts.

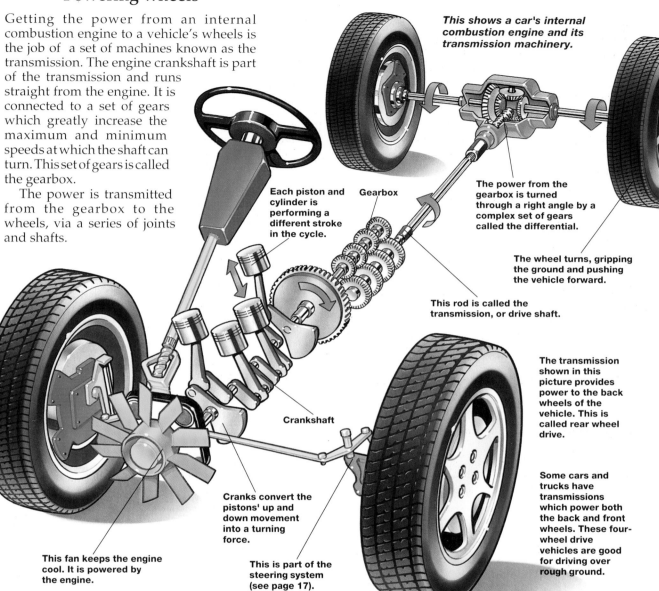

This shows a car's internal combustion engine and its transmission machinery.

Each piston and cylinder is performing a different stroke in the cycle.

Gearbox

The power from the gearbox is turned through a right angle by a complex set of gears called the differential.

The wheel turns, gripping the ground and pushing the vehicle forward.

This rod is called the transmission, or drive shaft.

The transmission shown in this picture provides power to the back wheels of the vehicle. This is called rear wheel drive.

Some cars and trucks have transmissions which power both the back and front wheels. These four-wheel drive vehicles are good for driving over rough ground.

Crankshaft

Cranks convert the pistons' up and down movement into a turning force.

This fan keeps the engine cool. It is powered by the engine.

This is part of the steering system (see page 17).

How many cylinders?

Many simpler machines, such as early motorcycles and some lawn mowers, run on one cylinder, but others have many more. The power in a single cylinder engine is provided by the third stroke of the engine's cycle. This means that the power is only provided once every four strokes. Most cars are powered by engines with four cylinders. So, at any one time, each cylinder is performing a different stroke. The more cylinders an engine has, the smoother and more continuous the power. Some sports and luxury car engines have as many as 12.

Pollution and other problems

Chemicals in the fuel that internal combustion engines use cause pollution. Pollution can damage both your health and the environment. In addition, the engine's fuel is produced by processing oil which only exists in limited quantities and is gradually being used up.

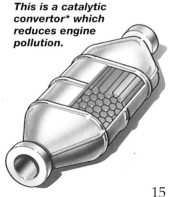

This is a catalytic convertor* which reduces engine pollution.

Land machines

The invention of the wheel and axle revolutionized the way people moved on land because it made possible the development of carts and carriages. Before they were invented, people walked on foot, carrying their own possessions or putting them on animals' backs.

Wheeled carts greatly increased the efficiency of load-carrying animals. The axle supported the load and the wheel reduced friction between the ground and the load. This meant that heavier loads could be moved at a faster speed and with much less effort than before.

The first mechanical vehicles

For many centuries, the most efficient land transport was provided by a cart or carriage pulled by an animal, such as a mule or a horse. In 1769, a French soldier named Nicholas Cugnot ran the first machine to move on land without an animal. His working steam tractor had a speed of about 4km/h (2mph).

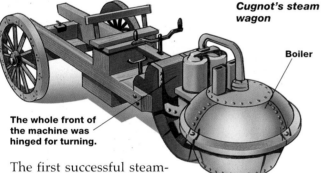

Cugnot's steam wagon

Boiler

The whole front of the machine was hinged for turning.

The first successful steam-powered train was built in 1804 by Richard Trevithick. The first commercial train service opened in Britain in 1825 between Stockton and Darlington. Railway lines soon spread across Europe, the United States and eventually throughout the world. Today, electrically-driven trains run efficiently at high speeds. It is not unusual to board a train which has an average speed of over 200km/h (115mph).

Motor vehicles powered by internal combustion engines weren't popular until the end of the 19th century. The first motor vehicles were nicknamed "horseless carriages". They were no faster or more comfortable than horse-drawn coaches. But improvements made between 1890 and 1930 led to the development of the sort of motor vehicle you are familiar with today.

The French TGV runs at speeds of up to 300km/h (180mph).

Machines within a machine

A modern motor vehicle is made up of many other machines, all of which have a special purpose. The central illustration shows a motorbike. It is powered by an internal combustion engine but it also contains other machines to make it easy to ride and control. Three of these components - steering, suspension and braking - are vital to any modern motor vehicle, whether it's a motorbike, car or truck.

This is a Ducatti M900 motorbike.

Steering

The motorbike on the right has a simple steering system, just like the one on a bicycle. Handlebars act as levers turning the motorbike's front wheel.

A modern car steering system is a little more complicated. It is based on a set of gears called a rack and pinion.

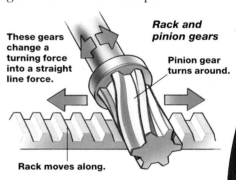

Rack and pinion gears

These gears change a turning force into a straight line force.

Pinion gear turns around.

Rack moves along.

A car steering wheel provides the initial turning force and is linked to the pinion gear. The pinion gear connects with a sliding toothed rail called a rack. As the pinion gear turns, it moves the rack along. The rack is joined to the wheel by track rods and steering arms, which point the wheels in one direction or another.

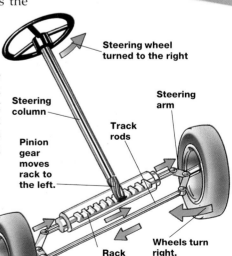

Steering wheel turned to the right

Steering arm

Steering column

Track rods

Pinion gear moves rack to the left.

A car's steering system

Rack

Wheels turn right.

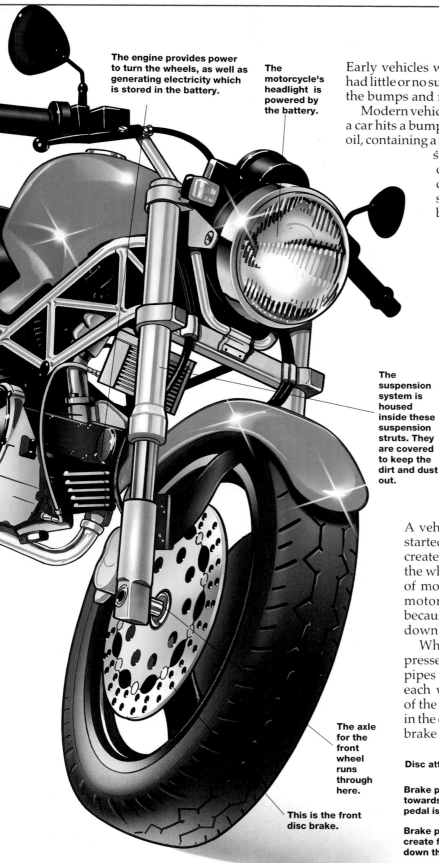

The engine provides power to turn the wheels, as well as generating electricity which is stored in the battery.

The motorcycle's headlight is powered by the battery.

The suspension system is housed inside these suspension struts. They are covered to keep the dirt and dust out.

The axle for the front wheel runs through here.

This is the front disc brake.

Suspension

Early vehicles were often very uncomfortable as they had little or no suspension to cushion passengers against the bumps and ruts in the old roads.

Modern vehicles have springs which compress when a car hits a bump, so absorbing the shock. A cylinder of oil, containing a moving piston, is employed to slow the spring's release. This cylinder is called a damper, or shock absorber. The damper absorbs much of the spring's energy and stops it from bouncing straight up.

How a damper works

Spring compressed by bump

Piston connected to spring

Cylinder full of oil

Spring tries to bounce back up quickly.

Piston rises slowly up through cylinder.

Spring's bounce is reduced.

Braking

A vehicle has to be able to stop once it has started moving. This is done by brakes which create vast amounts of friction to slow down the wheels. There are several different types of modern brakes. The brakes used on the motorcycle here are called disc brakes, because the friction used to slow the wheel down is applied to a metal disc.

When the brake pedal is pressed, fluid flows through pipes into cylinders beside each wheel. The pressure of the fluid forces a piston in the cylinder to push the brake pads on to the disc.

A disc brake

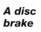

Disc attached to front wheel

Brake pads are pushed towards disc when brake pedal is pressed.

Brake pads grip disc hard and create friction which slows down the disc and the wheel.

Machines that float

All ships and boats, from the smallest dinghy to the largest oil tanker, rely on one thing: being able to float. Floating depends on both the weight and the size of an object. These are combined into a single measurement called density. Density can be measured in grams per cubic centimetre (g/cm^3), or in pounds per cubic foot (lbs/ft^3). Density is calculated by dividing an object's weight by its volume. The density of cold, fresh water is $1g/cm^3$. An object with less density floats; one with more density sinks.

This makes it easy to understand how light wooden boats float, but what about modern ships, which are mostly made of metal? The answer has to do with air, which is much less dense than water. Even the largest ocean liner is mostly made up of air. This makes the overall density of any boat, even when made with dense materials such as steel, less than water.

You can see this in practice by getting two equal-sized lumps of playdough. Drop the first one in some water. Its density is greater than water and it sinks. But then, shape a hollow boat out of the second lump and place it on the water. Because the volume of the boat contains a lot of air, its density is reduced to less than the density of water. As a result, it floats.

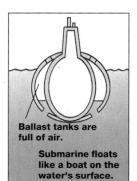

This log is less dense than water and so it floats.

Weight: 4000g or 8.8lbs
Volume: 8000cm or 0.28ft³
Density: 0.5g/cm³ or 31lbs/ft³

A density experiment

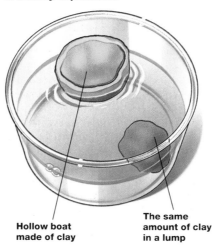

Hollow boat made of clay

The same amount of clay in a lump

This modern military submarine is just rising to the sea's surface.

This is the periscope. it allows the submarine crew to see above water while the craft is still just under the water.

Submarines

Submarines can vary their density so that they float either on top of the water, like a normal boat, or below the water. They manage to do this with the aid of huge containers in the submarine called ballast tanks. These are filled with either water or air. By varying the proportion of each substance in the tanks, the submarine can control its overall density and so determine whether or not it floats.

How a submarine dives and rises

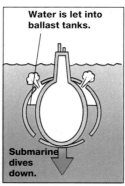

Ballast tanks are full of air.

Submarine floats like a boat on the water's surface.

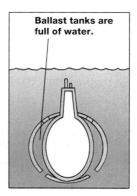

Water is let into ballast tanks.

Submarine dives down.

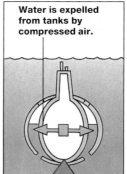

Ballast tanks are full of water.

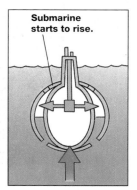

Water is expelled from tanks by compressed air.

Submarine starts to rise.

Powering floating machines

The earliest boats were rafts and dugout canoes, made from logs and powered by hand-held paddles. The paddles act as levers. The broad blade pushes the water back, forcing the boat forward. The next step was the introduction of sails to propel the boat by catching the wind.

Modern sails, based on the shape of the airfoil, enable ships to sail at an angle to the wind. With a zig-zagging movement called tacking, these vessels can even sail directly into the wind.

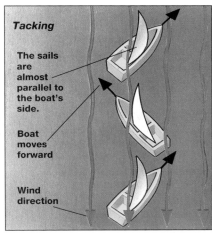

Tacking

The sails are almost parallel to the boat's side.

Boat moves forward

Wind direction

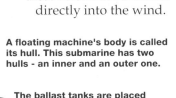

A floating machine's body is called its hull. This submarine has two hulls - an inner and an outer one.

The ballast tanks are placed between the two hulls.

The inner hull is where the crew live and work. It is called the pressure hull.

Submarines dive to great depths. The outer hull needs to withstand the great force of the sea pressing down upon it.

Propeller

Engines and propellers

Ships powered by steam engines first appeared in the 19th century. This meant that for the first time ships were able to travel without worrying about the wind. The first Atlantic crossing by a steamship was made in 1819 by an American craft called the *Savannah*.

These early steamers used their engines to drive a series of paddles shaped like water wheels. Paddles were soon replaced by a simple form of screw called a propeller. Today, most ships that don't use sails have internal combustion rather than steam engines, but they still use the engine to drive a propeller.

A ship propeller

Broad, curved blades

These are called hydroplanes. They act like aircraft wings and work with the ballast tanks to move the submarine up and down.

Cutting through water

Like all forms of transport, boats have to overcome friction. A boat must make the water in front of it move out of the way, before it can move forward. A hull with a wedge-shaped front reduces friction and allows the craft to move efficiently. Some boats, such as barges and oil tankers, do not need to travel fast. This sort of boat tends to have a flat-bottomed hull, which allows more cargo to be carried and makes the craft more stable.

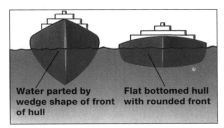

Water parted by wedge shape of front of hull

Flat bottomed hull with rounded front

Floating machines that fly

The drag created by water means that ordinary boats cannot obtain speeds much greater than 35km/h (20mph). But if a boat's hull is lifted out of the water in some way, the drag decreases and the speed can increase. This is what makes a speedboat move so quickly.

Among the fastest of all marine craft is the hydrofoil. A hydrofoil travels with its entire hull out of the water for most of the time. It moves on wing-like floats called foils, which are based on the airfoil. These provide the craft with lift and stability. The foils are much smaller than a boat's hull, which means that drag is reduced and speed increased.

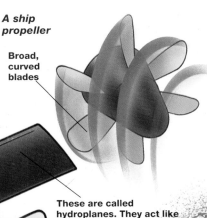

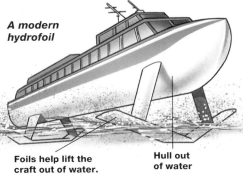

A modern hydrofoil

Foils help lift the craft out of water.

Hull out of water

Machines that fly

Moving in air is rather like moving in water. In both cases you have to stay "afloat". For a boat to float, it needs to have a hollow hull, making it less dense than water. In the same way, a machine that can float in air needs to be lighter than the air itself.

The very first machine to float in the air was the hot air balloon, first built in 1783 by two French brothers, the Montgolfiers. The invention of the airship (a balloon with an engine) 70 years later meant that for the first time a machine's flight could be controlled without worrying about the strength and the direction of the wind.

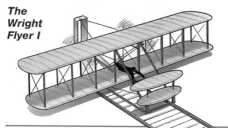

A modern balloon

But how can a hot air balloon float in air? The reason is that when air is heated, it expands. This means you don't need as much hot air to fill a balloon as you would cold air. As a result, the air inside the balloon is less dense than the air outside it. So, the balloon floats.

Heavier-than-air flight

Ever since ancient times, people have tried to build flying machines which were heavier than air. All attempts failed until the introduction of small engines, and wings based upon the airfoil principle.

The first heavier-than-air flying machine with an engine flew in 1903. It was built in the United States by the Wright brothers and had a small internal combustion engine which turned two propellers around.

The Wright Flyer I

Forces of flight

There are four forces involved in getting an aircraft off the ground and into the air. These are arranged in pairs called thrust and drag, and lift and gravity. Thrust is the force which tries to push the aircraft forward. It succeeds if it is greater than the drag, which is the friction that tries to slow the aircraft down.

To get an aircraft off the ground, you need enough lifting force to overcome the force of gravity. Lift is provided by the wings of a plane moving through the air. Aircraft wings are modelled on the shape of the airfoil.

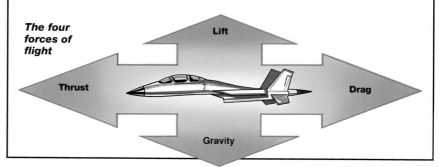

The four forces of flight

Controlling a plane

An aircraft's direction is altered by the hinged parts of the wing, called ailerons, and the hinged parts of the tail, called the elevators and rudder. Known collectively as control surfaces, these are simple wedges which deflect the air that flows past them. They are moved by two levers found in the cockpit, called the control column and the rudder bar.

In gliders and light aircraft, the cockpit controls are linked to the control surfaces by a system of cables and pulleys. In bigger aircraft, *hydraulic power** or a small electric motor assists the process. In some modern aircraft, 'fly by wire' is used. This is a system whereby a computer sends signals along electrical wires to motors in the wing and tail.

The control surfaces

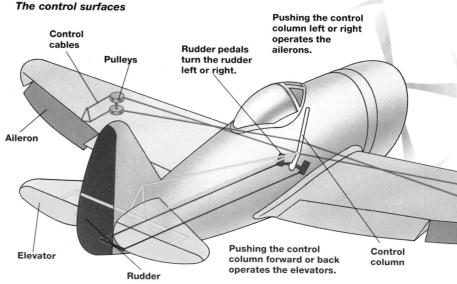

Control cables

Pulleys

Aileron

Elevator

Rudder

Rudder pedals turn the rudder left or right.

Pushing the control column left or right operates the ailerons.

Pushing the control column forward or back operates the elevators.

Control column

Directions of movement

An aircraft uses its control surfaces to move in a combination of three different directions. These are called roll, pitch and yaw.

A propeller-driven aircraft may have an internal combustion engine similar to a car engine.

An aircraft propeller needs to push great amounts of air back to pull the plane through the air.

Moving the plane's nose up or down is called pitching. It is controlled by the aircraft's elevators.

This direction of movement is called rolling. It is controlled by the aircraft's ailerons.

An aircraft's propeller blades are long and thin, so that they can cut through the air.

Aileron

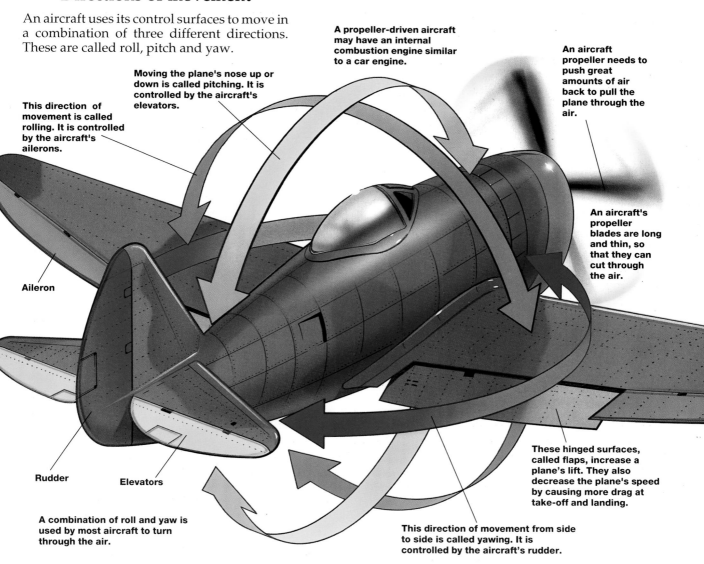

Rudder

Elevators

These hinged surfaces, called flaps, increase a plane's lift. They also decrease the plane's speed by causing more drag at take-off and landing.

A combination of roll and yaw is used by most aircraft to turn through the air.

This direction of movement from side to side is called yawing. It is controlled by the aircraft's rudder.

Elevators and rudder in action

You can see how elevators and ailerons work by making a simple paper plane. Tear the same sized flap in the back of each wing. These flaps work like elevators. Make a small tail out of thin cardboard and glue it to the back of the plane. Tearing a flap into the tail makes the rudder. Bending the elevators up causes the plane to climb. Bending the rudder in one direction causes the plane to go in that direction.

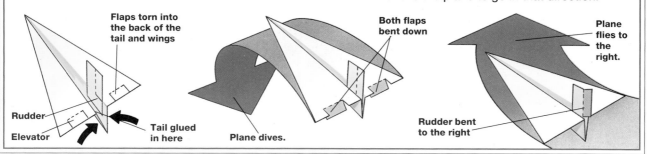

Flaps torn into the back of the tail and wings

Rudder

Elevator

Tail glued in here

Both flaps bent down

Plane dives.

Plane flies to the right.

Rudder bent to the right

Machines in space

Getting a machine into space isn't easy. That is why it didn't happen until long after machines were moving on water, land and air. A spacecraft has to be launched with enough speed to break away from the Earth's strong gravity. At first, scientists thought they would be able to fire a machine into space just as a cannon fires a cannonball. But after much research and many test flights, they realized that the best way was to put an engine on the spacecraft, so that it could move away from Earth under its own power.

Rocket engines

Modern spacecraft all use rocket engines. The rocket works on the principle that a force in one direction causes an equal force in the opposite direction. This is known as the *action-reaction** principle.

A rocket burns fuel in a combustion chamber which has an open end called a nozzle. As the fuel burns, it creates rapidly expanding gases which rush out of the exhaust. The strong downward force of the escaping gases is matched by an equally strong force in the opposite direction, which pushes the rocket up.

As a rocket heads up through the Earth's thinning *atmosphere**, it finds less oxygen to burn in its engines. So the rocket has to carry not only the engine and fuel, but also its own oxygen supply. Many rockets solve this by being divided into a number of stages, each with its own engine. Once a stage has run out of fuel (as shown here), it can be dropped off. This decreases the rocket's weight.

Make a balloon rocket

You will need a long balloon, a piece of string, a straw, some clear adhesive tape and a clip. Blow up the balloon and close the end with the clip. Now thread the string through the straw and tape the straw to the balloon. Attach the string to a doorway, or get a friend to hold one end up as high as possible. Keeping the string taut, and with the balloon at the bottom, release the clip. Your balloon will fly up the string until it runs out of air.

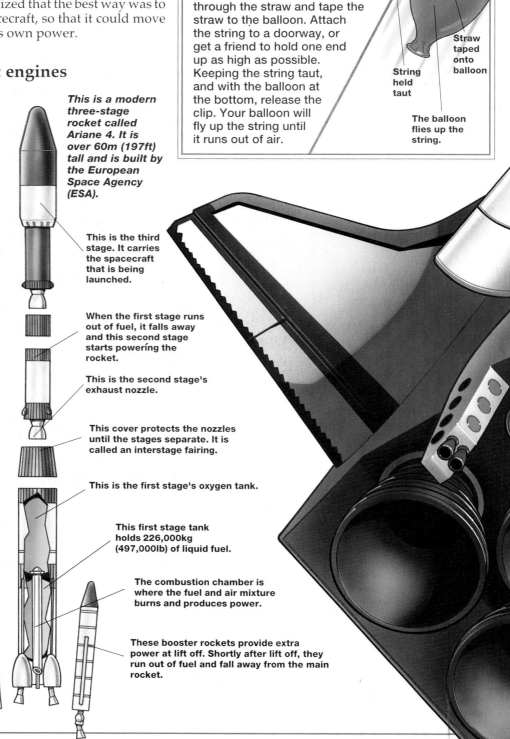

Straw taped onto balloon

String held taut

The balloon flies up the string.

This is a modern three-stage rocket called Ariane 4. It is over 60m (197ft) tall and is built by the European Space Agency (ESA).

This is the third stage. It carries the spacecraft that is being launched.

When the first stage runs out of fuel, it falls away and this second stage starts powering the rocket.

This is the second stage's exhaust nozzle.

This cover protects the nozzles until the stages separate. It is called an interstage fairing.

This is the first stage's oxygen tank.

This first stage tank holds 226,000kg (497,000lb) of liquid fuel.

The combustion chamber is where the fuel and air mixture burns and produces power.

These booster rockets provide extra power at lift off. Shortly after lift off, they run out of fuel and fall away from the main rocket.

Space shuttles

The space shuttle is powered by engines similar to those found in an ordinary rocket. It is different, however, because it provides a reusable method of launching spacecraft. The shuttle is streamlined to overcome the great amounts of friction it encounters on leaving Earth's atmosphere. Once in space, atmospheric friction is unimportant and the shuttle can release unstreamlined spacecraft into orbit.

The space shuttle, built in the United States, made its first spaceflight in 1981.

The shuttle's robot arm can extend out some 15m (51.7ft). It can position objects to within 5cm (2").

The shuttle's cargo bay can hold up to 29,500kg (64,900lb) of satellites or experiments.

A craft that is launched into space by a rocket or shuttle is called the payload.

The shuttle has wings and a tail like an ordinary aircraft. These help it glide back down to Earth after it has completed its mission.

The shuttle has two smaller rocket engines which help it change direction once in space.

The three main rocket engines propel the shuttle into space.

This satellite is called the Long Duration Exposure Facility (LDEF). It contains lots of experiments, including the measurement of space radiation.

Satellites

Although the most famous space events, such as landing on the moon, used manned spacecraft, the majority of machines in space are unmanned spacecraft called satellites. Satellites constantly fall around the curve of the Earth, in a process called orbiting.

The very first satellite, the Russian *Sputnik 1*, was also the first man-made object in space. Since then, over 5000 satellites have been launched. A number of satellites are used to collect information about the Earth. These satellites take photographs or create *radar** images of the Earth's surface and its atmosphere for use in weather forecasting, mineral exploration and agriculture.

Returning to Earth

The Earth's gravity helps a spacecraft orbit around the planet. It also helps a spacecraft return to Earth. If the orbiting speed of a spacecraft is reduced sufficiently, the Earth's gravity will take effect and the spacecraft will spiral down to Earth. As the spacecraft enters the Earth's upper atmosphere, the friction of the air both slows down the craft and heats it up. Many unmanned spacecraft are left to burn up and fall apart in the atmosphere. But the space shuttle (right) is designed to glide down to Earth. It has special insulating outer layers, which prevent the craft from burning up during re-entry.

Outer surface glows red hot during re-entry.

Time machines

Machines that tell the time are something we take for granted today, but reasonably accurate clocks and watches did not exist until a few hundred years ago. Up till then, people used a number of ways of telling the time, none of which were very reliable. For example, the rising and setting sun provided a rough guide, but only when the weather was clear. Water clocks and hourglasses filled with sand measured the time it took a substance to flow out of a hole in a container. These were more accurate, but not practical for longer periods.

The first reliable clocks were not built until the 13th and 14th centuries. These were mechanical devices driven by a slowly falling weight, but they were not accurate enough to have a minute hand. Clocks greatly improved in the 17th century with the introduction of two things: the pendulum and escapement.

The pendulum and escapement

A pendulum is a free-swinging object which has a back and forth motion. The important thing about it is that the time it takes to move through an arc is not dependent on the angle of the swing, but on the length of the pendulum itself. An individual pendulum will always take the same length of time to complete a swing.

The principle of the pendulum was first discovered in 1581 by the Italian scientist, Galileo. The first pendulum clock was built in the 1650s by the Dutch scientist, Christian Huygens.

The pendulum is linked to a mechanism called an escapement, which gradually, and at regular intervals, releases the weight that powers the clock. There are many different types of escapement. One of the most common ones is an anchor escapement, shown on the left. The escapement has two toothed ends called pallets. They engage with a geared wheel called an escape wheel.

The anchor escapement

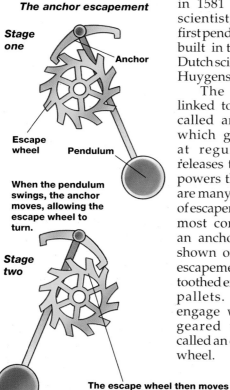

Stage one

Anchor

Escape wheel

Pendulum

When the pendulum swings, the anchor moves, allowing the escape wheel to turn.

Stage two

The escape wheel then moves one notch before being stopped by the anchor.

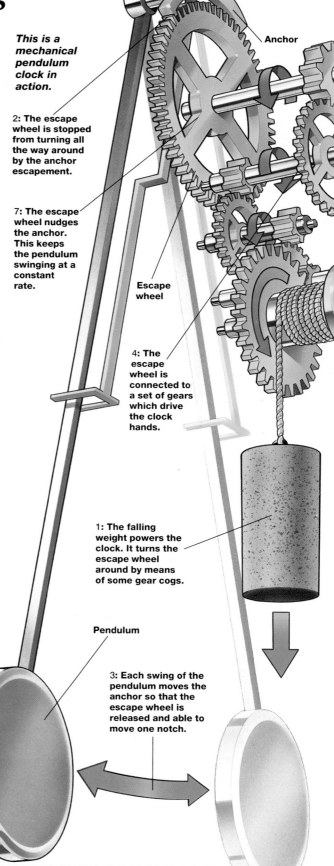

This is a mechanical pendulum clock in action.

Anchor

2: The escape wheel is stopped from turning all the way around by the anchor escapement.

7: The escape wheel nudges the anchor. This keeps the pendulum swinging at a constant rate.

Escape wheel

4: The escape wheel is connected to a set of gears which drive the clock hands.

1: The falling weight powers the clock. It turns the escape wheel around by means of some gear cogs.

Pendulum

3: Each swing of the pendulum moves the anchor so that the escape wheel is released and able to move one notch.

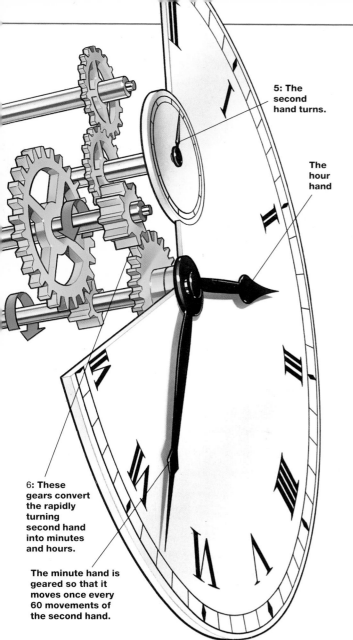

5: The second hand turns.

The hour hand

6: These gears convert the rapidly turning second hand into minutes and hours.

The minute hand is geared so that it moves once every 60 movements of the second hand.

Springs

Later, mechanical clocks were powered by springs, instead of a falling weight. The advantage of a spring was that once wound up tightly, it could release its energy in regular, controlled amounts. This enabled accurate watches to be made for the first time.

The very first watch, made by German locksmith Peter Heinlein in 1500, used a strip spring to power it. Soon, some mechanical clocks and most watches had two springs: a mainspring for power and a coiled spring, called a hairspring, to regulate movement.

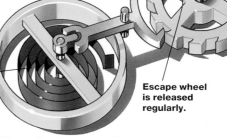

A hairspring

Hairspring gradually unwinds.

Escape wheel is released regularly.

Vibrating crystals

The mineral quartz has properties which make it vibrate at a very fast and regular rate when an electric current is applied to it. This vibration, known as the piezo-electric effect, can be used to produce an incredibly accurate signal at regular intervals. This signal was first used to control a tiny motor which turned the hands and gears of a quartz clock or watch. In modern digital watches, however, the vibration is used to power an electronic circuit rather than mechanical gears.

Inside a digital watch

Circuit

Time display

Battery

The most accurate clocks in the world

Technology has moved on so much this century that clocks can now be made that are accurate to an incredible one second every 1.7 million years. These clocks use individual atoms which vibrate like quartz, but at a much faster rate. The first atomic clock used atoms of a chemical called cesium and was completed in 1955.

Another development designed to increase accuracy is taking place high up in space. Launched in 1988, the Laser Synchronization from Stationary Orbit (LASSO) project synchronizes atomic clocks all around the world.

The Meteosat satellite containing the LASSO project

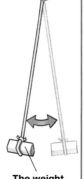

Making a pendulum

You can make a pendulum with an eraser and a piece of string just over 1m (40") long. Tie the string firmly around the eraser. Then hold the string tightly so that there is about 90cm (36") free to swing. Raise the eraser so that the string is parallel to the ground, and let it swing. Notice how the swings get shorter and shorter. But even though they are all of a different size, you will find that each swing will take about one second.

The weight on the end is called a bob.

The human machine

A sports car, a screwdriver and a human being: which is the odd one out? The answer is none of them, because they are all machines. The human body is not a single machine, like a screwdriver. It is more like a sports car: a collection of machines. Often these machines work together. For example, your front teeth act as wedges cutting through food when you bite. Your jaw increases the force with which your teeth can bite. It acts as a lever as you open and close your mouth.

Wedge-shaped tooth drives into food.

Wedge pushes food apart as it cuts.

Muscles and bones

Your body contains over 200 bones, connected to a large number of muscles. These provide most of your body's movement.

A single muscle can only contract and pull part of your body. For that part of your body to move from one position and then back to its original position, there needs to be another, opposing muscle pulling in the opposite direction.

Arms act as levers. The upper arm muscles (biceps and triceps) provide the effort to lift the load which is carried in the hand. The elbow is the pivot point.

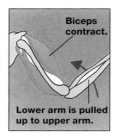

Biceps contract.

Lower arm is pulled up to upper arm.

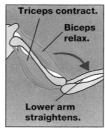

Triceps contract.

Biceps relax.

Lower arm straightens.

Body breakdown

Just like a bicycle or a car, your body can also break down if it isn't looked after. Some of the problems it faces are the result of friction.

Lubrication is one way of reducing friction. You oil your bicycle to make its parts move more easily and to reduce wear and tear on those parts. Many of your joints are lubricated in a similar way.

A human knee joint

Femur

Tibia

Synovial capsule contains lubricating fluid which reduces the friction of bones rubbing together.

Cartilage cushions your leg bones from damage as they bump and rub together.

Your body's limits

The human body is a very effective machine. Even with modern advances in technology, it is still better at performing some tasks than man-made mechanical devices. For example, your hands can do a far wider variety of tasks than the best mechanical claw.

But your body does have limits too, and this is where machines are very useful. Some machines can help a person perform tasks in situations that would be dangerous or impossible for a human being. The solid-bodied diving suit shown on the right is one such example.

This special diving suit is a complex extension to the human body. Called a JIM suit, it enables divers to stay underwater for long periods of time.

This backpack has two propellers powered by small engines. These help propel the diver around the sea bed.

Body repair

As medical science has improved, it has become possible to replace more and more parts of the body which are defective, or have suffered too much wear. Some replacement parts, such as kidneys, are transplants from other people's bodies. But many others, including artificial limbs, heart valves and hip bones are man-made.

A modern artificial hand

Hand's electronics linked to a tiny computer

Jointed fingers

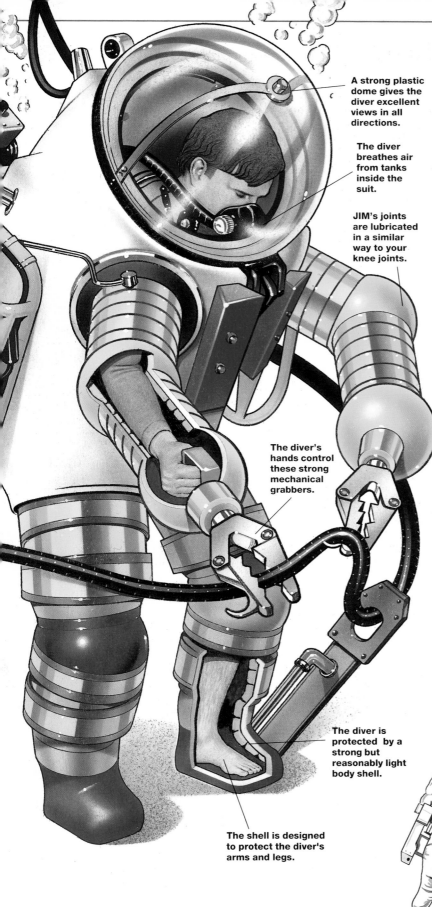

A strong plastic dome gives the diver excellent views in all directions.

The diver breathes air from tanks inside the suit.

JIM's joints are lubricated in a similar way to your knee joints.

The diver's hands control these strong mechanical grabbers.

The diver is protected by a strong but reasonably light body shell.

The shell is designed to protect the diver's arms and legs.

Machines as extensions

Many everyday machines do things which people can do themselves. They act as an extension to the person, helping him or her to perform the task more easily. For example, you can try to draw a circle freehand, but a pair of compasses will help you draw a far more accurate circle.

An Archimedes screw is an efficient way of pumping water out of a river or lake.

Handle turned

Water pumped out here

Water drawn off by screw

Sport and lever extensions

Many simple extensions are levers. For example, a crowbar is a lever which enables you to exert more force when opening a door or crate. Many sports rely on machines which act as lever extensions to the human body. Golf clubs and baseball bats are both levers, enabling players to get more force or distance into their shots or hits.

The length of a tennis racket acts as a lever, increasing the force hitting the tennis ball.

The handle and head of the racket increases the distance a player can reach.

Man amplifiers

One of the most advanced types of extension is the man amplifier. This machine forms an external skeleton, called an exoskeleton, around a person's body. Man amplifiers can exert greater force on objects than the human body can by itself. Man amplifiers can also protect a person from powerful and dangerous forces.

This man amplifier is called a Manned Maneuvering Unit. Astronauts use it for moving around in space.

Robots and automation

Automatic machines are all around you, from cash-dispensers outside banks, to microwaves in the home. An automatic machine is one which can perform a task with little human intervention. In some cases, automatic machines have replaced the work of humans, because machines can be stronger, faster, more convenient and more efficient.

Some automatic machines are made of materials that are more resistant to damage than the human body. This means that they can operate in dangerous environments, for example, in a radiation-filled nuclear reactor, or at the bottom of the ocean.

Early automatic machines

The first automatic machines date back as early as the Middle Ages. They were hinged metal figures found on large mechanical clocks. A system of gears within the clock made sure that the figures struck the clock's bell at a specific time.

From the 18th century, mechanical puppets appeared which mimicked human actions. They were called automatons and were often built by very highly skilled clock and watchmakers.

This Swiss automaton, just 26cm (10") high, can write short sentences.

During the industrial revolution, many factory machines were produced which required little more than a supervisor to check that the machine was working properly. But these machines could only perform one fixed task. The French weaver Joseph-Marie Jacquard (1752-1834) made a major breakthrough by building a loom that could be programmed to carry out different commands.

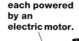

Jacquard's loom accepted cards punched with holes as the instructions for the pattern that it should weave.

Robots

The invention and development of the electronic computer has made possible a range of machines which can be easily programmed. Today, there are programmable machines called robots which have the ability to react to their environment and any changes that occur within it.

Modern industrial robots are extremely useful for performing simple, repetitive tasks (the sort of tasks that a person would soon get very bored and careless with over time). Another advantage of industrial robots is that, apart from occasional interruptions for maintenance, they can work around the clock, greatly increasing production.

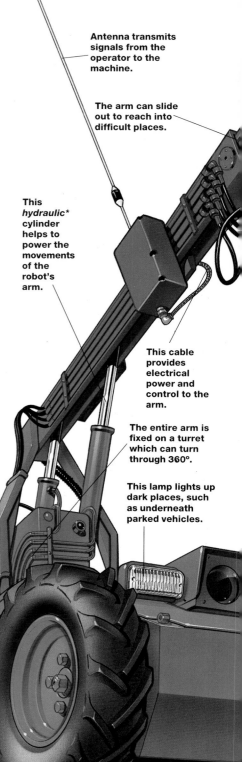

Antenna transmits signals from the operator to the machine.

The arm can slide out to reach into difficult places.

This *hydraulic** cylinder helps to power the movements of the robot's arm.

This cable provides electrical power and control to the arm.

The entire arm is fixed on a turret which can turn through 360°.

This lamp lights up dark places, such as underneath parked vehicles.

This is a remote-controlled bomb disposal machine. The operator remains a safe distance away from the unexploded bomb.

The machine moves on six wheels, each powered by an electric motor.

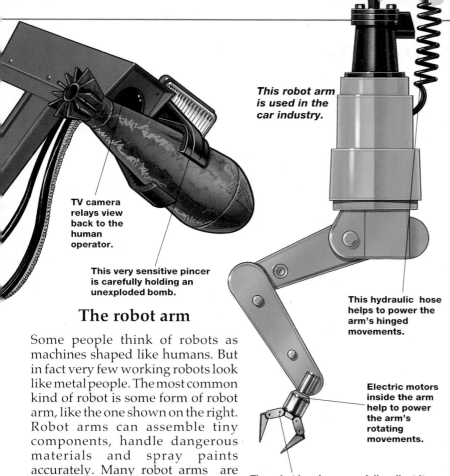

TV camera relays view back to the human operator.

This very sensitive pincer is carefully holding an unexploded bomb.

This robot arm is used in the car industry.

This hydraulic hose helps to power the arm's hinged movements.

Electric motors inside the arm help to power the arm's rotating movements.

The robot hand can carefully adjust its grip to hold anything, from a fine piece of wire to a heavy car engine part.

The robot arm

Some people think of robots as machines shaped like humans. But in fact very few working robots look like metal people. The most common kind of robot is some form of robot arm, like the one shown on the right. Robot arms can assemble tiny components, handle dangerous materials and spray paints accurately. Many robot arms are powered by a combination of *hydraulics** and electric motors.

Directions of movement

Robots can move in a number of directions. Each one is called a degree of freedom. A robot arm tends to have up to six degrees of freedom. Three of these come from the wrist joint, which allows movement in three possible directions - twisting around (known as roll), side-to-side (yaw), and up and down (pitch).

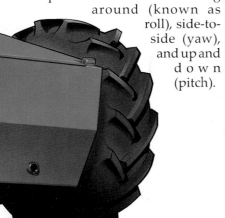

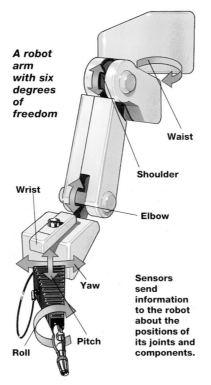

A robot arm with six degrees of freedom

Waist

Shoulder

Wrist

Elbow

Yaw

Roll

Pitch

Sensors send information to the robot about the positions of its joints and components.

Some amazing robots

This research robot made by the University of Bristol in England can play snooker or pool. It works out the angles and force of shot needed.

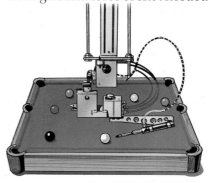

"Sim one" is a medical robot, which responds to treatments like a human patient. It is used to train doctors and nurses.

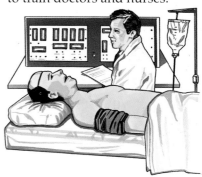

The Cybermotion SR2 robot acts as a security guard. It patrols large buildings at night.

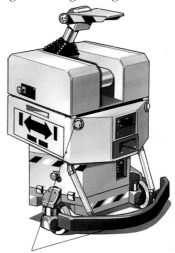

This robots's sensors can trace movement and detect intruders.

Looking into the future

A hundred years ago, there were no aircraft, space rockets or computers. No one knows what kinds of machines there will be in the future, but several general predictions can be made.

It is likely that some established machines, such as engines and planes, will continue to be developed and improved. Some forms of transport will become faster and offer more facilities to the passenger.

Computers will be used more and more to design and build machines. Computers will also be increasingly found inside machines to control them. Some industrial machines may get bigger while a number of others, including robots, will get smaller for use in medicine and other fields.

More efficiency, less pollution

Vast quantities of resources, such as metals and *fossil fuels**, are used to build and run machines. Many of these resources are already beginning to run out. Another drawback is that machines cause pollution, which damages the environment. To combat these problems, machines are increasingly being designed to be more efficient, use fewer resources and create less pollution.

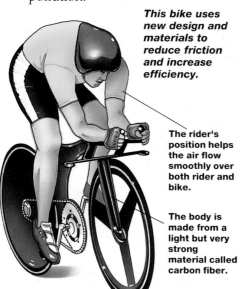

This bike uses new design and materials to reduce friction and increase efficiency.

The rider's position helps the air flow smoothly over both rider and bike.

The body is made from a light but very strong material called carbon fiber.

Magnetic levitation

Mechanical parts suffer more from friction and tend to be more expensive to make than electronic ones. So in the future it is likely that, where possible, scientists and engineers will use fewer mechanical components and more electronic ones. One example of this, the Magnetic Levitation (Maglev) train, is already in existence. To see how it works, try placing the north *poles** (or south poles) of two magnets together and watch how they push apart. Maglev trains work on the same principle, but with enormously powerful magnets. These lift the train up and keep it hovering no more than 10cm (4") above the ground. With no touching surfaces between train and ground, friction is greatly reduced. It also means that fewer mechanical parts are needed.

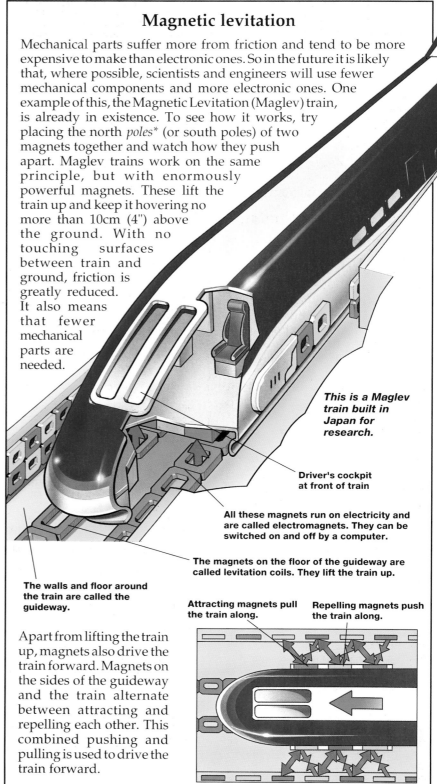

This is a Maglev train built in Japan for research.

Driver's cockpit at front of train

All these magnets run on electricity and are called electromagnets. They can be switched on and off by a computer.

The magnets on the floor of the guideway are called levitation coils. They lift the train up.

The walls and floor around the train are called the guideway.

Attracting magnets pull the train along.

Repelling magnets push the train along.

Apart from lifting the train up, magnets also drive the train forward. Magnets on the sides of the guideway and the train alternate between attracting and repelling each other. This combined pushing and pulling is used to drive the train forward.

Did you know...?

One of the smallest motors in the world is this one built by Toshiba. It is tiny and uses very little power, but turns at a speed of up to 10,000 revolutions per minute.

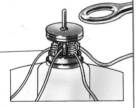

The motor measures less than 1mm (0.04") across.

Intermediate technology

Complex machines tend to use more resources than simple ones, as well as being harder to repair. In some situations, an old, simple machine can do a job just as well as a more complicated modern model.

These sorts of issues have led to the development of a set of ideas known as intermediate technology. One of its main principles is that a machine should be tailored to individual requirements. Where possible, it should be made from local materials and should not damage the environment. It should also be powered by an energy source under the control of the local population. For example, a simple archimedes screw might be ideal as a water pump in the desert, whereas an electric pump might easily clog with sand, break down and have to be sent a long way away to be fixed.

This simple, bicycle-powered trailer is built and used by local people in Sri Lanka. It is called a Cartitt.

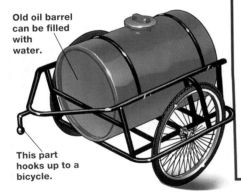

Old oil barrel can be filled with water.

This part hooks up to a bicycle.

Glossary

Here is a short list explaining some of the more complicated terms found in this book. When a word appears in *italics*, it has its own entry in the list.

Action-reaction. A law of physics which states that forces always occur in pairs. Whenever one force occurs, there is also an equal but opposite force. This second force is called the reaction force.

Airfoil. An object shaped to produce lift when air flows over or under it. This shape is most often seen in aircraft wings.

Atmosphere. The layer of gases that surrounds the Earth. Other planets have atmospheres made up of different gases.

Axle. A bar or rod on which a gear or a wheel, turns.

Catalytic convertor. A device which helps remove some of the harmful substances from an engine's waste gases.

Compound machine. A machine consisting of two or more simple machines.

Cylinder. A hollow tube in an engine in which a *piston* can move up and down.

Density. The measurement of how much of a substance is present in a given *volume*.

Differential. A set of gears that allow the powered wheels of a motor vehicle to turn at different speeds when the vehicle goes around a corner.

Energy. The capacity of something to move or change. Energy can also be described as the ability to do *work*.

Force. A pulling or pushing action which produces change or movement.

Fossil fuels. Fuels formed from animal and vegetable matter which is compressed over many millions of years, in the same way that fossils are created. The world's industry at the moment depends on fossil fuels. Natural gas, coal and oil are all examples of fossil fuels.

Friction. The resistance found when one surface moves and rubs against another surface.

Geothermal power. The heat energy which is produced by natural processes inside the Earth. It can be extracted from hot springs, reservoirs of hot water deep below the ground or by breaking open the rock itself.

Gravity. The force of attraction that pulls all objects together. This force is not noticeable unless one or both objects are very large, like the Earth or another planet.

Hydraulic. A hydraulic machine is one that is operated by a compressed liquid which produces a strong force over a short distance. Early hydraulic machines, such as cranes, used water, but most hydraulic machines today use oil or other liquids that do not freeze as easily as water.

Igniting. Setting fire to something, such as the fuel and air mixture found in a car engine. In a car engine, the parts which start burning the fuel and air mixture are called the ignition system.

Internal combustion engine. A type of engine in which fuel is burned inside a cylinder which moves a piston up and down.

Jet engine. A type of engine which provides thrust forward by pushing great amounts of air and other gases out behind.

Liquid crystal display (LCD). Made of special crystals which react to electricity, an LCD shows the numbers on most calculators, digital watches and some portable computers.

Lubrication. Covering surfaces that rub together with a slippery liquid which helps to reduce friction.

Piston. A device which fits inside a cylinder and moves up or down.

Pivot point. The point about which a lever turns. When an arm acts as a lever and lifts something, the elbow is the pivot point.

Pneumatic. A pneumatic machine is one that is operated by a compressed gas, usually air. Some trucks' suspension systems run on compressed air.

Poles. The end of a magnet is called its pole.

Power. The speed or rate at which energy is produced, supplied or used.

Pressure. The force with which one object presses upon another. It is often used in terms of the force that a liquid or gas presses on an object, as in air pressure (see page 13).

Radar. A system using signals called radio waves to detect moving objects, particularly aircraft, in the sky.

Streamlining. To shape an object in a way that makes it move as smoothly as possible through air or water. The more easily a vehicle can move, the less power it has to use.

Volume. A measurement of how much space an object occupies. Volume is measured in cubic centimetres or cubic inches.

Work. The amount of effort used to perform a task. Work is measured in joules.

Index

Many thanks to:

Dr. Ed Abel, British Hovercraft
Corporation Ltd., Central Japan Railway
Co., Cybermotion, Intermediate
Technology, Liebharr GB Ltd., Martin
Marietta, NASA, Unimation Ltd., UNIMEX
Handels Gmbh., Westland Aerospace

First published in 1993 by Usborne Publishing,
83-85 Saffron Hill, London EC1N 8RT, England.
First published in America in August 1994.
All rights reserved. No part of this publication
may be reproduced, stored in a retrieval
system, or transmitted in any form, or by any
means, electronic, mechanical or otherwise,
without the prior permission of the publisher.

Copyright 1993 Usborne Publishing Ltd. The
name Usborne and the device 🐦 are Trade
Marks of Usborne Publishing Ltd. AE

Printed in Spain.